Clinical Guide to Popular Diets

Clinical Guide to Popular Diets

Edited by
Caroline Apovian
Elizabeth Brouillard
Lorraine Young

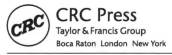

CRC Press
Taylor & Francis Group
Boca Raton London New York

CRC Press is an imprint of the
Taylor & Francis Group, an **informa** business

Cover design concept created by Mary-Catherine Stockman, RD, LDN

CRC Press
Taylor & Francis Group
6000 Broken Sound Parkway NW, Suite 300
Boca Raton, FL 33487-2742

Library of Congress Cataloging–in–Publication Data

Names: Apovian, Caroline M., editor. | Brouillard, Elizabeth, editor. | Young, Lorraine (Physician), editor.
Title: Clinical guide to popular diets / [edited by] Caroline Apovian, Elizabeth Brouillard & Lorraine Young.
Other titles: Popular diets
Description: Boca Raton : CRC Press, Taylor & Francis Group, 2018.
Identifiers: LCCN 2017048956 | ISBN 9781498774307 (pbk.)
Subjects: LCSH: Reducing diets--Evaluation.
Classification: LCC RM222.2 .C51945 2018 | DDC 613.2/5--dc23
LC record available at https://lccn.loc.gov/2017048956

Visit the Taylor & Francis Web site at
http://www.taylorandfrancis.com

and the CRC Press Web site at
http://www.crcpress.com

Contents

Introduction

As most clinicians know obesity rates continue to rise, with the most recent NHANES data, from 2011–2014, indicating that 36.5% of US adults are considered obese.[1] The health risks of obesity are well researched and documented, including type 2 diabetes, cardiovascular disease, hypertension, stroke, gallbladder disease, osteoarthritis, sleep apnea, and some types of cancer.[2] Modest weight loss of 5%–10% has been shown to significantly improve obesity-related conditions.[3] The physiology behind obtaining this weight loss is a negative energy balance, however, the diet macronutrient composition for the best results is still debated. The American Heart Association, American College of Cardiology, and The Obesity Society performed a systemic review of the literature and found that of the 17 diets with varying macronutrient composition that have been studied, no diet was superior for weight loss or weight maintenance. However, the biggest predictor of weight loss was determined to be adherence to a diet.[2] As a clinician, many patients may look to you to recommend a diet program. Since no one diet has demonstrated superiority, it is important to understand the available diet plans on the market in order to guide your patients to the diet right for them; one they will be able to incorporate into their lifestyle for long-term success.

This book will provide you with a non-biased review of several popular diets that have been available and marketed for many years. The diets in this review include The Atkins Diet, The DASH (Dietary Approaches to Stop Hypertension) Diet, the iDiet, the Mediterranean Diet, Paleo Diets, South Beach Diet, vegetarian diets, Weight Watchers, and the Zone Diet. Each chapter will give you an overview of the diet, explain how the diet works, provide current research, illustrate typical results, list the pros and cons of the diet, and suggest patients that would benefit most from each diet. Our goal with this book is to assist you in guiding your patients to choose a diet that is most appropriate for them and one they will be able to follow for long-term results.

REFERENCES

1. Centers for Disease Control and Prevention (CDC). National Center for Health Statistics (NCHS). *National Health and Nutrition Examination Survey Data.* Hyattsville, MD: U.S. Department of Health and Human Services, Centers for Disease Control and Prevention; 2016. https://www.cdc.gov/nchs/data/factsheets/factsheet_nhanes.htm
2. Jensen M, Ryan D. et al. 2013 AHA/ACC/TOS guideline for the management of overweight and obesity in adults. A report of the American College of Cardiology/American Heart Association. *J AM Coll Cardiol* 2014;63(25):2985–3023.
3. National Institutes of Health, National Heart, Lung, and Blood Institute. Obesity Education Initiative. Clinical guidelines on the identification, evaluation, and treatment of overweight and obesity in adults. *Obes Res* 1998;6(Suppl 2):51S–210S.

Editors

Caroline Apovian, MD, FACP, DABOM, is professor of Medicine and Pediatrics, in the Section of Endocrinology, Diabetes, and Nutrition at Boston University School of Medicine, USA. She is also director of the Center for Nutrition and Weight Management at Boston Medical Center, USA. Dr. Apovian is a nationally and internationally recognized authority on Nutrition and Obesity Medicine and has been in the field of Obesity and Nutrition since 1990. Her current research interests are in: weight loss and its effects on endothelial cell function obesity and cardiovascular disease, adipose cell metabolism and inflammation, resolution of diabetes and cardiovascular disease in the bariatric surgery population, disparities in the treatment of obesity in underserved populations, and novel pharmacotherapeutic anti-obesity agents. She is also an expert in the technique for subcutaneous adipose tissue biopsies, and has been studying the relationship between adipose tissue inflammation and obesity for over 10 years. Dr. Apovian was a member of the expert panel for updating the 2013 AHA/ACC/TOS Clinical Guidelines for the Management of Overweight and Obesity in Adults, published in *Circulation and Obesity* journals and was the Chair of the Endocrine Society guidelines for Medical Treatment of Obesity published in the *Journal of Endocrinology and Metabolism* in 2015.

Dr. Apovian was a recipient of the Physician Nutrition Specialist Award given by the American Society of Clinical Nutrition. This was for her work on developing and providing nutrition education to medical students and physicians in training at Boston University School of Medicine. She has published over 200 original peer-reviewed articles, chapters, and reviews on the topics of: obesity, nutrition, and the relationship between adipose tissue and risk of developing cardiovascular disease.

Dr. Apovian has given over 150 invited lectures nationally and internationally and currently serves as President Elect of The Obesity Society (TOS) for 2016-17.

Elizabeth Brouillard, RD, LDN, CDE, is the Nutrition Manager for The Center of Endocrinology, Diabetes, Nutrition and Weight Management at Boston Medical Center. She completed her dietetic degree at the University of Maryland and went to New Presbyterian Hospital for her clinical internship. She has been a registered dietitian for 10 years and has focused most of her career on weight management and diabetes. She obtained a certificate in adult weight management from the Academy for Nutrition and Dietetic and is a Certified Diabetes Educator. Elizabeth works in outpatient settings and sees patients every day struggle to make diet and lifestyle changes for weight loss and glycemic control. Many of her patients have tried several different diets with varying success in the past and Elizabeth has been able to work with these patients to determine which diet plan will work best for them based on their current health, lifestyle, and food preferences.

Lorraine Young, RD, MS, CNSC, LDN, is the Clinical Nutrition Manager (CNM) and Home Nutrition Support Dietitian at Boston Medical Center (BMC). This position is part of the Department of Endocrinology, Diabetes and Nutrition. She is also an Instructor of Medicine at Boston University School of Medicine. She is responsible for the management of all in-patient Clinical Nutrition Services and dietitians for both adult and pediatric patients as well as two pediatric outpatient dietitians. Clinically, she manages all home parenteral and complex enteral patients discharged from the hospital or referred to the Endocrinology, Diabetes and Nutrition Department, which includes many short bowel patients and patients with Inflammatory Bowel Disease.

She has over 35 years of experience in the field of Nutrition Support as well as in conducting clinical research with one of the original developers of parenteral nutrition in the United States. These research projects included work with intravenous and enteral glutamine and growth hormone in critically ill patients. She also manages complex bariatric surgery patients who may have developed complications and may require specialized nutrition therapies. She is a co-investigator on an NIH funded R21 to study the Effects of Metabolic Support immediately post-trauma with Dr. Peter Burke, Director of BMC's Trauma Center. She has been involved as a consultant in an International Research Program with AFINS project (Abbott Fund in Nutritional Sciences) whose goal is to improve inpatient Clinical Nutrition Services in Vietnam. She has published extensively with over 50 publications in the clinical nutrition field. She was the first recipient of the Dietitian's in Nutrition Support Research Award and was also a recipient of the Massachusetts Young Dietitian Award in the 1980s. As the CNM at the hospital, she also serves as a teacher, lecturer, and mentor to the hospital nutrition and medical staff.

Contributors

Laura Andromalos
Clinical Nutrition
Virginia Mason Medical Center
Seattle, Washington

Meghan Ariagno
General and GI Surgery
Brigham and Women's Hospital
Boston, Massachusetts

Megan Barnett
Department of Endocrinology, Weight
    Management, and Nutrition
Boston Medical Center
Boston, Massachusetts

Caroline Blanchard
Energy Metabolism Laboratory
Jean Mayer USDA Human Nutrition
    Center on Aging
Tufts University
Boston, Massachusetts

Sai Krupa Das
Energy Metabolism Laboratory
Jean Mayer USDA Human Nutrition
    Center on Aging
Tufts University
Boston, Massachusetts

Catherine Fanning
Nutrition Boston Medical Center
Boston, Massachusetts

Madeleine M. Gamache
Energy Metabolism Laboratory
Jean Mayer USDA Human Nutrition
    Center on Aging
Tufts University
Boston, Massachusetts

Glenn K. Harvin
Division of Gastroenterology,
    Hepatology and Nutrition
Brody School of Medicine
East Carolina University
Greenville, North Carolina

Micaela C. Karlsen
Nutritional Epidemiology
    Laboratory
Jean Mayer USDA Human Nutrition
    Center on Aging
Tufts University
Boston, Massachusetts

Amy Krauss
Energy Metabolism Laboratory
Jean Mayer USDA Human Nutrition
    Center on Aging
Tufts University
Boston, Massachusetts

Laura E. Matarese
Division of Gastroenterology,
    Hepatology and Nutrition
Brody School of Medicine
East Carolina University
Greenville, North Carolina

Thomas J. Moore
Boston University School of
    Medicine
University in Boston
Boston, Massachusetts

Megan Murphy
e-Havior Change, LLC
Waban, Massachusetts

Lin Pao-Hwa
Department of Medicine
Nephrology Division
Duke University Medical
    Center
Durham, North Carolina

Susan B. Roberts
Energy Metabolism Laboratory
Jean Mayer USDA Human Nutrition
    Center on Aging
Tufts University
Boston, Massachusetts

1 The Atkins Diet

Laura E. Matarese and Glenn K. Harvin

CONTENTS

OVERVIEW

Despite the fact that there are well over 1000 published weight-loss diets in the lay literature, few have attracted as much attention as the Atkins Diet. The late Dr. Robert C. Atkins developed this low-carbohydrate, high-protein weight-loss plan which was publicized in his best-selling book, *The Atkins Diet Revolution.*[1] Dr. Atkins promoted the plan as not only a quick weight-loss diet but as a change in eating for a lifetime. The diet was extremely popular allowing individuals to consume large quantities of meat and high-fat foods without considering caloric restrictions. Critics referred to the diet as a high-protein, high-fat, low-carbohydrate ketogenic diet which could be potentially harmful. Early claims on both sides were often fueled by perception and personal biases without scientific evidence. Eventually, the emergence of numerous clinical trials appeared in the scientific literature demonstrating the efficacy and safety of the Atkins Diet.

HOW THE DIET WORKS

Historically, obesity has been considered to be a result of an imbalance in caloric intake versus expenditure. The idea was simple: when individuals take in more calories than they expend, the result will be weight gain. Given the growing incidence of obesity worldwide, however, it has become clear that this represents an over-simplification of a complex disease whose cure is more complicated than simply creating a caloric deficit. Physiologically, carbohydrate restriction, as opposed to a negative energy balance, is responsible for initiating the metabolic response to fasting.[2] The Atkins hypothesis is that dietary carbohydrate, particularly from simple sugars, causes hyperinsulinemia, leading to insulin resistance, obesity, and the metabolic syndrome. Excess carbohydrate prevents effective lipolysis with resulting lipogenesis. Low carbohydrate diets reduce the dietary contribution to serum glucose thereby lowering insulin levels. Insulin is a potent stimulator of lipogenesis and inhibitor of lipolysis. Lowering insulin levels allows the utilization of stored body fat for energy. Severe carbohydrate restriction leads to a progressive depletion of glycogen stores eventually switching metabolism to lipolysis. With a reduction in dietary carbohydrate, there is a corresponding increase in dietary protein and fat. This leads to the production of ketones which act as an appetite suppressant and contribute to an overall voluntary caloric reduction.[3,4] It has been proposed that inefficient protein and fat oxidation leads to additional energy loss since more adenosine triphosphate (ATP) is required to oxidize these macronutrients.[5] Lipolysis is maintained despite excess calories because glycerol from fat is needed as a gluconeogenic precursor.[2] The carbohydrate level required to produce the metabolic shift from lipogenesis to lipolysis has been debated, but it is thought to be between 20 and 50 g of carbohydrate per day in the initial phases of the diet. This contrasts sharply with the typical carbohydrate content of the Western diet which often exceeds 300 g per day comprising large quantities of simple, rapidly hydrolyzed carbohydrates.

THE ATKINS PLAN

The foundation of the Atkins Plan is a reduction of carbohydrates. The diet has evolved over the years to currently offer two options (Table 1.1). With Atkins 20™, the starting point (Phase 1, Induction) is 20 g of "Net Carbs" (carbohydrate minus grams of fiber) per day. The Atkins 40™ allows a starting point of 40 g of Net Carbs per day. Both plans allow for an increase in carbohydrates. One plan adds foods one at a time and the other raises the carbohydrate portion-size allowance as individuals approach their weight loss goals (Table 1.1).

The Atkins 20™ (the original plan) includes a four-step process beginning with a two-week induction phase with carbohydrates restricted to 20 g Net Carbs per day (Table 1.2). The carbohydrates are derived primarily from low-glycemic, nutrient-dense, fiber-rich carbohydrates such as leafy green salads and other non-starchy vegetables. The client is instructed to consume 4–6 oz. of protein at each meal and enough natural fat to feel satiated. *Trans* fats are eliminated. The protein is derived from a variety of sources to include meat, fish, poultry, eggs, and vegetable-based proteins such as tofu. Adequate fluid (water preferred) intake along with exercise and a complete multivitamin/mineral supplement is recommended in order to obtain optimal nutrition. Dairy intake is limited because of its carbohydrate content, therefore, calcium supplementation is recommended.

The second phase of the program is referred to as the ongoing weight loss phase. During this phase, carbohydrates are added into the diet in the form of

TABLE 1.1

Comparison of the Atkins Diet Plans

	Atkins 20™	Atkins 40™
	Initial Phase of Weight Loss	
Net carbs (grams)	20	40
Protein	3 servings of 4–6 oz per serving	3 servings of 4–6 oz per serving
Healthy fats	3 servings of added healthy fats per day, e.g., butter, salad dressings, olive oil, etc.	3 servings of added healthy fats per day, e.g., butter, salad dressings, olive oil, etc.
Carbohydrates	Limited—Most carbs are derived from vegetables during first 2 weeks, e.g., leafy greens and other low-carb vegetables Dairy foods high in fat and low in carbs: cream, sour cream, and most hard cheeses are allowed	All Food Groups—About 1/3 carbs from vegetables, remaining carbs from fruit, nuts, and/or whole grains
Phase 2 of weight loss increasing carbohydrates	Add in 5 g net carb increments starting with lower carb foods and gradually progressing to higher carb foods • Nuts and seeds (but not chestnuts) • Berries, cherries, and melon (but not watermelon) • Whole milk yogurt and fresh cheeses, such as cottage cheese and ricotta • Legumes, including chickpeas, lentils, and the like • Tomato and vegetable juice "cocktail" • Other fruits (but not fruit juices or dried fruits) • Higher-carb vegetables, such as winter squash, carrots, and peas	Add 10 g of net carbs when individual is within 10 pounds of goal weight by increasing serving size or adding more variety 10 g of net carbs may be added each week as long as weight loss continues. Continue to use the same acceptable foods list
	Weight Maintenance Phase	
Adding foods back into the diet	Progressive—Carbohydrates are slowly added back into the diet	All Food Groups—The acceptable foods list remains the same until goal weight is achieved
Protein	3 servings of 4–6 oz per serving	3 servings of 4–6 oz per serving
Healthy fats	3 servings of added healthy fats per day, e.g., butter, salad dressings, olive oil, etc.	3 servings of added healthy fats per day, e.g., butter, salad dressings, olive oil, etc.
Increasing carbohydrates	Carbohydrates are added back in 5 g net carb increments until weight stabilizes. That carb intake is continued to maintain weight	Carbohydrates are added back in 10 g net carb increments until weight stabilizes. That carb intake is continued to maintain weight

TABLE 1.2
Example Menu for Atkins 20™

	Breakfast	Net Carbs (g)
Phase 1—Induction		
Net carbs = 20 g/day	2 scrambled eggs (with milk)	2.0
	1/2 medium tomato	2.0
	1/2 Haas avocado	1.5
	Coffee/tea	0
	Snack	
	String Cheese, 1 oz.	1.0
	Cucumber, 1/2 cup	1.6
	Lunch	
	1 cup mixed greens	1.5
	Grilled chicken	0
	Caesar Dressing	1.0
	Coffee/tea/water/diet soda	0
	Snack	
	2 celery stalks	2.0
	Creamy Italian dressing	2.0
	Coffee/tea/water/diet soda	0
	Dinner	
	Grilled salmon	0
	Steamed broccoli (1/2 cup)	2.2
	Arugula salad (1 cup)	0.4
	Coffee/tea/water/diet soda	0
	Total net carbs	17.2
Phase 2—Ongoing Weight Loss		
Net carbs start at 25 g/day gradually increasing intake in 5 g increments each week or every several weeks until weight loss ceases or begins to slow. Net carb prescription is then reduced by 5 g.	Yellow squash and Gruyere frittata	2.5
	Coffee/tea	0
	Snack	
	2 tablespoons oil roasted mixed nuts	2.0
	Coffee/tea/water/diet soda	0
	Lunch	
	Canned tuna	0
	1/4 cup red bell pepper	1.5
	1/2 medium tomato	2.0
	Coffee/tea/water/diet soda	0
	Snack	
	4 oz. whole milk Greek yogurt	6.1
	1/2 cup fresh blackberries	3.3

(Continued)

TABLE 1.2 (*Continued*)
Example Menu for Atkins 20™

	Breakfast	Net Carbs (g)
Dinner		
Flank steak		0
Grilled asparagus (6)		2.0
1 cup Romaine hearts		1.0
2 tablespoons Green Goddess dressing		1.0
1/2 cup fresh raspberries		3.4
Total net carbs		24.8

Phase 3—Pre-Maintenance		
Carbohydrate intake increased by 10-gram increments every week to maintain very gradual weight loss, generally half a pound a week. Once the goal weight is achieved, the individual remains at that carbohydrate intake level until body weight stabilizes for one month.	*Total net carbs*	Variable

Phase 4—Lifetime Maintenance		
Emphasis on sustainable changes to lifestyle in order to maintain the weight loss. Individuals continue to eat the same variety of foods as in the last month of Pre-Maintenance, while controlling carbohydrate intake to ensure weight maintenance. Since body fat is no longer the primary source of energy, a slightly greater intake of natural fats is necessary to maintain weight.	*Total net carbs*	Variable

nutrient-dense, fiber-rich foods increasing to 25 g of Net Carbs per day during the first week. The carbohydrate content is further increased each week or every several weeks in 5-gram increments until weight loss ceases or begins to slow. At this point, the Net Carb prescription is reduced by 5 g. The individual remains at this level for a sustained, moderate weight loss, generally averaging one to two pounds per week.

Phase three is "Pre-Maintenance," which transitions the individual from weight loss to weight maintenance by increasing daily carbohydrate intake in 10-gram increments every week for several weeks to maintain very gradual weight loss, generally half a pound a week. Once the goal weight is achieved, the individual remains at that carbohydrate intake level until body weight stabilizes for one month.

The final phase is referred to as "Lifetime Maintenance." Emphasis is placed on sustainable lifestyle changes in order to maintain the lower weight. Individuals continue to eat the same variety of foods as in the last month of Pre-Maintenance while controlling carbohydrate intake to ensure weight maintenance. A slight increased intake of natural fats is necessary to maintain the lower weight since body fat is no longer the primary source of energy.

Over the years, the diet has evolved to emphasize healthy protein and fat choices from a variety of foods. Vegetables are included in every phase of the Atkins program including the most restrictive induction phase. As an individual progresses through the diet phases, ingestion of more vegetables along with low-glycemic fruits, nuts, seeds, whole grains, and legumes is encouraged. Later versions of the original Atkins Diet acknowledged that exercise is important for weight loss and maintenance as well as for achieving overall health benefits.

CURRENT RESEARCH

Designing controlled trials to evaluate the safety and efficacy of dietary interventions is challenging. Randomization of interventions is possible, but blinding is difficult. Results may vary depending on whether the study was conducted as an outpatient in a "free-living" environment versus a controlled metabolic inpatient setting. The study population may not always be homogenous in terms of the disease process, comorbidities, age, gender, body mass index (BMI), and medications. Adherence to a dietary intervention is not always optimal, making interpretation of the results difficult. Outcome parameters vary considerably and many are poorly defined. For example, it may be debated whether weight loss alone is an adequate outcome parameter or whether it is more important to look at changes in risk factors for disease and medication requirements. Many studies were underpowered, short in duration, or had high dropout rates, leading investigators to perform meta-analyses. There is a significant body of literature despite these challenges that has evaluated the low-carbohydrate Atkins Plan. Many of the studies evaluated the "low carbohydrate" concept, but the actual study design may or may not necessarily follow the "Atkins Diet." For the purpose of this review, all studies evaluating low carbohydrate diets are considered to be indicative of the Atkins Diet.

EFFECTS OF CARBOHYDRATE RESTRICTION FOR INDIVIDUALS WITH TYPE 2 DIABETES AND METABOLIC SYNDROME

Diabetes is a disease of altered carbohydrate metabolism. There are a number of factors which increase the risk of type 2 diabetes. Individuals who are overweight or obese, especially central obesity, can have insulin resistance. Obesity, in addition to high blood pressure, high cholesterol, and triglycerides, results in metabolic syndrome. It is logical to assume that reduction of dietary carbohydrate content may result in better glucose management and weight loss.

Feinman and colleagues' systematic review concluded that dietary carbohydrate restriction should be the first approach in diabetes management.[5] Restriction of dietary carbohydrate consistently reduces elevated blood glucose independent of weight loss, and reduces the requirement of medications to control blood sugar such as insulin. There is also evidence that improved glucose concentrations, weight loss, and lipid profiles reduce the cardiovascular risk seen in individuals with type 2 diabetes.

If dietary carbohydrate restriction is beneficial for individuals with type 2 diabetes, what is the optimal level of restriction to achieve these beneficial effects? Westman and colleagues randomized 84 subjects with obesity and type 2 diabetes to receive either a low-carbohydrate, ketogenic diet or a low-glycemic index diet over a 24-week trial.[6] The low-carbohydrate group lost more weight (11.1 kg) compared to the low-glycemic group (6.9 kg). The hemoglobin A1c was reduced by 1.5% in the low-carbohydrate group compared to 0.5% in the low-glycemic group. Diabetes medications were either reduced or eliminated in 95.2% of the low-carbohydrate group compared to 62% in the low-glycemic group, and only the low-carbohydrate group achieved an increase in high-density lipoprotein (HDL) cholesterol.

Since individuals with diabetes often have significant cardiovascular risk profiles, Tay and colleagues compared the effects of a very-low-carbohydrate, high-unsaturated fat, low-saturated fat (LC) diet with a high-carbohydrate, low-fat (HC) diet on glycemic control and cardiovascular disease risk factors in 115 obese patients with type 2 diabetes over a 52-week trial.[7] Both diets were hypocaloric. The LC diet provided 14% of energy as carbohydrate (50 g/d), 28% of energy as protein, and 58% of energy as fat (10% saturated fat). The energy-matched, HC diet provided 53% of energy as carbohydrate, 17% of energy as protein, and 30% of energy as fat (10% saturated fat). Both groups received supervised aerobic and resistance exercise for 60 minutes, three days per week. Study completion rates were similar in both groups as were weight loss, blood pressure, HbA1c, and reduction in fasting glucose. The LC diet, however, which was high in unsaturated fat and low in saturated fat, achieved greater improvements in the lipid profile, blood glucose variability, and reductions in diabetes medication requirements.

Samaha and colleagues randomized 132 severely obese subjects (mean BMI, 43 kg/m^2), many of whom had metabolic syndrome or type 2 diabetes, to either an ad libitum low-carbohydrate, ketogenic diet (LCKD) or a calorie-restricted, low-fat diet (LFD).[8] The study was conducted in an ambulatory setting and subjects received weekly group counseling sessions for four weeks followed by monthly sessions. At six months, there was significantly greater weight loss (5.8 kg vs 1.9 kg; P = 0.002) and triglyceride reduction (20% vs 4%; P = 0.001) in the LCKD group compared with the LFD group. Diabetic subjects in the LCKD group demonstrated improved serum glucose (decrease of 25 mg/dL versus a decrease of 5 mg/dL; P = 0.01) compared with their LFD group, whereas the nondiabetic subjects in the LCKD had improved insulin sensitivity (6% vs −3%; P = 0.01) compared with their LFD group. Seven LCKD subjects had a reduction of diabetic medication dosage compared with only one from the LFD group. Overall, the low-carbohydrate diet resulted in significantly more beneficial effects on body weight and metabolic parameters.

There have been a number of these individual trials in subjects with type 2 diabetes. A systematic review and meta-analysis of the dietary approaches to the management of type 2 diabetes was conducted by Ajala and colleagues.[9] A total of 20 randomized controlled trials (RCTs) with 3073 patients were included in final qualitative analyses and 16 studies were included in the quantitative analysis. The low carbohydrate, low-glycemic index, Mediterranean, and high-protein diets all led to a greater improvement in glycemic control with HbA1c reductions compared with their respective control diets. The largest effect was seen in the Mediterranean Diet. The low-carbohydrate and Mediterranean Diets led to greater weight loss of more than 20 kg and an increase in HDL seen in all diets except the high-protein diet. Overall, the data suggests that controlling carbohydrate intake, particularly of simple sugars, results in better blood sugar control, weight loss, and even reduction in diabetic medications.

EFFECTS OF CARBOHYDRATE RESTRICTION ON CARDIOVASCULAR DISEASE

Obesity and dyslipidemia are modifiable factors associated with cardiovascular disease. There has been a concern that the high-protein/low-carbohydrate diets which are high in fat may lead to an increase in blood cholesterol, triglycerides, and low-density lipoproteins. To evaluate the effects of diet on weight loss and lipid profiles, Aude and colleagues randomized 60 overweight subjects to receive the low-fat National Cholesterol Education Program (NCEP) diet or a diet that was low in carbohydrate and high in monosaturated fat over a 3-month period.[10] Both groups received a caloric restriction. Weight loss was significantly greater in the low-carbohydrate group (6.2 kg) compared to the NCEP group (3.4 kg), (P = 0.02). There were no significant differences between the groups for total, low density, or high density lipoprotein cholesterol, triglycerides, or the proportion of small, dense, low-density lipoprotein particles. The low-carbohydrate group did show a significant reduction in triglycerides. Waist-to-hip ratio was not significantly reduced between the groups (P = 0.27), but it significantly decreased within the low carbohydrate group (P = 0.009).

Volek and colleagues conducted a detailed analysis of the effects of dietary intervention on weight loss and metabolic and lipoprotein markers.[11] Forty overweight subjects with dyslipidemia were randomized to a low-carbohydrate diet or a low-fat diet over a 12-week period. Both diets were energy-restricted and overall caloric intake was similar for both groups. Each of the dietary interventions resulted in improvements in metabolic parameters. The low-carbohydrate group had reduced glucose (−12%) and insulin (−50%) concentrations, insulin sensitivity (−55%), weight loss (−10%), and decreased adiposity (−14%). The low-carbohydrate group also demonstrated a more favorable lipid profile including a reduction of triacylglycerol (−51%) and increase in HDL cholesterol (13%) and total cholesterol/HDL-cholesterol ratio (−14%) response. The low-carbohydrate diet also demonstrated positive effects on other cardiovascular risk factors including postprandial lipemia (−47%), Apolipoprotein B/Apolipoprotein A-1 ratio (−16%), and low-density lipoprotein (LDL) particle distribution. The saturated fatty acids in the triacylglycerols and cholesteryl esters and palmitoleic acid were significantly decreased in the low-carbohydrate group compared to subjects consuming the low-fat diet.

Foster and colleagues studied the effects of targeted diet interventions on weight loss and lipid profiles over the course of one year.[12] Sixty-three subjects were randomized to receive a low-fat, calorie-restricted diet or a low-carbohydrate diet without a caloric restriction. The low-carbohydrate group experienced greater weight loss (7.3% vs 4.5%) and improvements in triglycerides and HDL compared to the low-fat group. This study demonstrated that it was the composition of the macronutrients as opposed to energy that influenced weight loss and changes in lipid profiles.

Yancy and colleagues conducted a number of studies to evaluate the effects of LCKD in overweight and obese individuals with dyslipidemia. In one study, the ad libitum LCKD along with vitamin supplementation was compared to a low-fat, low cholesterol, reduced-calorie diet. LCKD participants followed the traditional Atkins Diet using an unrestricted energy intake with initial carbohydrate restriction to less than 20 g per day.[13] Carbohydrates were gradually increased as goal body weight was approached. Completion of the trial was greater in the subjects on the LCKD compared to the reduced-calorie subjects (75% versus 53%; P = 0.03). Weight loss was greater in the LCKD subjects compared to the low-fat subjects (14% reduction versus 9% reduction; P < 0.001). The LCKD group also demonstrated beneficial changes in serum lipids with a decrease in triglycerides of 42% and increase in HDL cholesterol by 13%. There was not a significant change in total cholesterol and LDL cholesterol. Their data were corroborated in another trial in which ambulatory overweight subjects with hyperlipidemia were randomly assigned to LCKD (<20 g), (N = 59) or a low-fat (<30%), low-cholesterol, reduced-calorie diet (n = 60) for 24 weeks.[14] Both groups received exercise and participated in group meetings. The low-carbohydrate group lost more weight, had higher HDL-C levels, and had a greater reduction in triglyceride levels.

There have been numerous trials which have looked at the effects of low-carbohydrate diets on weight loss and lipid profiles. A systematic review of randomized controlled trials of the LC diets versus low fat from 2000 to 2007 showed that the low-carbohydrate, high-protein diet was more effective at six months and was as effective if not more so as the low-fat diet in reducing body weight and cardiovascular risk parameters up to 1 year.[15] Several other systematic reviews with meta-analyses have been conducted on the low-carbohydrate, ketogenic diet versus the low-fat diet. In each of these analyses, the low-carbohydrate diet produced greater weight loss and improved cardiovascular risk parameters.[16–19]

WEIGHT LOSS, COMPLIANCE, AND RECIDIVISM

In both short to medium term studies, low-carbohydrate, high-protein diets have resulted in greater weight loss compared to high-carbohydrate, low-fat diets. The degree of weight loss may have varied, but overall, the low-carbohydrate diets produce greater weight loss compared to the low-fat diets. In most of the studies, calories were restricted in the low-fat groups, while subjects in the low-carbohydrate group enjoyed an unrestricted caloric intake with an overall emphasis on macronutrient content. In those studies which had caloric restriction for both groups, the low-carbohydrate diets resulted in greater weight loss,[11,20] although this was not the case in some of the studies.[21–23] In one study of subjects with type 2 diabetes, the low-fat group lost more weight (0.5 kg) than the low-carbohydrate group, but the results were not statistically significant.[24] In those studies which evaluated the change in visceral fat, the low-carbohydrate diets demonstrated greater reduction.[10,11] Brehm and colleagues demonstrated a reduction in body fat as measured by DXA in healthy women with a very low-carbohydrate diet compared with a low-fat group at three and six months.[25]

Compliance with any dietary intervention or plan is always a concern with adherence often decreasing over time. In those studies reporting this data, non-compliance occurred with both the low-carbohydrate and the low-fat diets. There was a slight compliance advantage overall with the low-carbohydrate diet. The reason may be that the low-carbohydrate diet was associated with reduced appetite.[26,27]

The ability to maintain the weight loss declines in both groups, but there appears to be a slight advantage with the low-carbohydrate plan. The Atkins Plan is a lifestyle plan designed to help individuals lose weight and maintain that weight loss. Individuals that abandon the overall plan after achieving their desired weight loss and return to their previous eating habits will regain their weight.

TYPICAL RESULTS

As with any weight-loss diet, individual results may vary. In general, healthy weight loss is considered to be two pounds per week. The initial weight loss on the Atkins Diet is dramatic and averages 8–15 pounds in the first two weeks. However, this initial weight loss is most likely due to a reduction in total body water and glycogen and not necessarily adipose tissue. Eventually, metabolism shifts to lipolysis and lean muscle is preserved. Some individuals with type 2 diabetes will experience a dramatic improvement and resolution of their diabetes when there is sufficient weight loss. Other comorbidities such as hypertension are generally improved as well. As a result, medications to control these conditions will have to be adjusted.

PROS AND CONS

The benefit of the Atkins Diet is that it results in dramatic reduction in body weight and often with reversal of comorbidities, improvement of lipid profiles, and reduction or elimination of associated medications. The Atkins Diet has a very good safety profile with extremely low reported complications. There are some potential complications that should be considered, nonetheless. The effects of low-carbohydrate, high-protein diets on urinary stone formation have not been extensively studied, and there are conflicting results.[28] There are some data to suggest that high-carbohydrate diets, especially from simple carbohydrates such as glucose or xylitol, result in an increase in calciuria.[29,30] Xylitol consumption has been associated with a rise in urinary excretion of phosphate and oxalate, which can promote the formation of calculi.[30] A high sucrose intake was associated with an increased risk for kidney stones in individuals with no history of kidney stones in the Nurses' Health Study.[31] Sucrose has been shown to result in increases in serum insulin and urine calcium excretion.[32] Although the data is limited, studies such as these would suggest that high-protein, low-carbohydrate diets are protective against renal stones.

One short-term study specifically addressed the effects of consumption of a high-protein, low-carbohydrate diet on kidney stone formation. This study showed a marked increase in the acid load to the kidney with an increased risk for stone formation and a decreased estimated calcium balance.[33] Thus, the exact effects of high-protein, low-carbohydrate diets on nephrolithiasis remain unclear.

Overall, reported complications are low, not serious, and generally from a few select case reports. Nevertheless, there are certain groups of individuals who may require additional monitoring or slight modifications to the Atkins Diet plan. For example, individuals with compromised renal function should be closely monitored or placed on a modified regimen that would not adversely affect renal function. Individuals with gout who become symptomatic should be placed on the maintenance phase of the program. Pregnant women and nursing mothers are advised to follow the maintenance phase of carbohydrate restriction, avoiding ketosis as a precaution. There is one reported case of ketoacidosis associated with a low-carbohydrate diet in a non-diabetic lactating woman.[34] However, her estimated carbohydrate intake was less than 20 g per day for 10 days prior to admission to the hospital, an amount that is even less than what is typically prescribed in the induction phase. The low-carbohydrate, high-fat diet in combination with the high substrate demand of lactation appears to be the etiology of this rare case of ketoacidosis.

IS THIS DIET RIGHT FOR YOU?

The diet has a very good safety profile. However, there are certain considerations that may influence the decision to embark on this dietary regimen. First, can you drastically reduce the carbohydrate and sugar in your diet including grains, fruit, and dairy products? The diet works by restricting grams of carbohydrates so the individual must be willing to calculate and keep track of the carbohydrate intake. Next, can you consume a high percentage of protein from meat, poultry, fish, eggs, and fats? If you are vegetarian, can you consume nuts, tofu and soy products, eggs, and cheese? Can you consume at least eight cups of water daily? Whether you are vegetarian or consume animal products, all individuals should take a multivitamin to ensure adequate intake of all micronutrients.

CONCLUSION

In each of these well-controlled clinical trials and meta-analyses, the low-carbohydrate ketogenic diet demonstrated superior weight loss when compared to more traditional approaches. There are some potential adverse effects, although they have not been observed in any of the clinical trials to date. These include the development of kidney stones, hypokalemia and hypomagnesaemia, elevated fatty acids, and gout in susceptible individuals. When this diet technique is employed in individuals taking medications for diabetes mellitus or hypertension, meticulous monitoring is required in order to prevent hypoglycemia and hypotension as body weight is rapidly reduced. Ultimately, the best weight-reduction diet is the one an individual will follow to achieve and maintain a healthy body weight.

REFERENCES

1. Atkins RC. *Dr. Atkins Diet Revolution*. New York: Bantam Books; 1972.
2. Kirk E, Reeds DN, Finck BN. et al. Dietary fat and carbohydrates differentially alter insulin sensitivity during caloric restriction. *Gastroenterology* 2009;136:1552–1560.
3. Boden G, Sargrad K, Homko C. et al. Effect of a low-carbohydrate diet on appetite, blood glucose levels, and insulin resistance in obese patients with type 2 diabetes. *Ann Intern Med* 2005;142:403–411.
4. Gibson AA, Seimon RV, Lee CMY. et al. Do ketogenic diets really suppress appetite? A systematic review and meta-analysis. *Obes Rev* 2015;16:64–76.

5. Feinman RD, Pogozelski WK, Astrup A. et al. Dietary carbohydrate restriction as the first approach in diabetes management: Critical review and evidence base. *Nutrition* 2015;31:1–13.

6. Westman EC, Yancy WS, Mavropoulos JC. et al. The effect of a low-carbohydrate, ketogenic diet versus a low-glycemic index diet on glycemic control in type 2 diabetes mellitus. *Nutr Metab* 2008;5(36):1–9.

7. Tay J, Luscombe-Marsh ND, Thompson CH. et al. Comparison of low- and high-carbohydrate diets for type 2 diabetes management: A randomized trial. *Am J Clin Nutr* 2015;102:780–790.

8. Samaha FF, Iqbal N, Seshardi P. et al. A low-carbohydrate as compared with a low-fat diet in severe obesity. *N Engl J Med* 2003;348:2074–2081.

9. Ajala O, English P, Pinkney J. Systematic review and meta-analysis of different dietary approaches to the management of type 2 diabetes. *Am J Clin Nutr* 2013;97:505–516.

10. Aude YW, Agatston AS, Lopez-Jimenez F. et al. The national cholesterol education program diet vs a diet lower in carbohydrates and higher in protein and monounsaturated fat. *Arch Intern Med.* 2004;164:2141–2146.

11. Volek JS, Phinney SD, Forsythe CE. et al. Carbohydrate restriction has a more favorable impact on the metabolic syndrome than a low fat diet. *Lipids* 2009;44:297–309.

12. Foster GD, Wyatt HR, Hill JO. et al. A randomized trial of a low-carbohydrate diet for obesity. *N Engl J Med* 2003;348:2082–2090.

13. Hickey JT, Hickey L, Yancy WS. et al. Clinical use of a carbohydrate-restricted diet to treat the dyslipidemia of the metabolic syndrome. *Metab Syndr Relat Disord* 2004;1(3):227–232.

14. Yancy WS, Olsen MK, Guyton JR. et al. A low-carbohydrate, ketogenic diet versus a low-fat diet to treat obesity and hyperlipidemia: A randomized, controlled trial. *Ann Intern Med.* 2004;140(10):769–777.

15. Hession M, Rolland C, Kulkarni U. et al. Systematic review of randomized controlled trials of low-carbohydrate vs. low-fat/low-calorie diets in the management of obesity and its comorbidities. *Obes Rev* 2009;10:36–50.

16. Bezerra Bueno N, Vieira de Melo IS, Lima de Oliveira S. et al. Systematic review with meta-analysis very-low-carbohydrate ketogenic diet v. low-fat diet for long-term weight loss: A meta-analysis of randomised controlled trials. *Br J Nutr* 2013;110:1178–1187.

17. Santos FL, Esteves SS, da Costa Pereira A. et al. Systematic review and meta-analysis of clinical trials of the effects of low carbohydrate diets on cardiovascular risk factors. *Obes Rev* 2012;13:1048–1066.

18. Hu T, Mills KT, Yao L. et al. Effects of low-carbohydrate diets versus low-fat diets on metabolic risk factors: A meta-analysis of randomized controlled clinical trials. *Am J Epidemiol.* 2012;176(Suppl):S44–S54.

19. Clifton PM, Condo D, Keogh JB. Long term weight maintenance after advice to consume low carbohydrate, higher protein diets—A systematic review and meta-analysis. *Nutr Metab Cardiovasc Dis* 2014;24:224–235.

20. Halyburton AK, Brinkworth GD, Wilson CJ. et al. Low- and high-carbohydrate weight-loss diets have similar effects on mood but not cognitive performance. *Am J Clin Nutr* 2007;86(3):580–587.

21. Meckling KA, O'Sullivan C, Saari D. Comparison of a low-fat diet to a low-carbohydrate diet on weight loss, body composition, and risk factors for diabetes and cardiovascular disease in free-living, overweight men and women. *J Clin Endocrinol Metab* 2004;89:2717–2723.

22. Tay J, Brinkworth GD, Noakes M. et al. Metabolic effects of weight loss on a very-low-carbohydrate diet compared with an isocaloric high-carbohydrate diet in abdominally obese subjects. *Am Coll Cardiol* 2008;51:59–67.

23. Brinkworth GD, Noakes M, Buckley JD. et al. Long-term effects of a very-low-carbohydrate weight loss diet compared with an isocaloric low-fat diet after 12 mo. *Am J Clin Nutr* 2009;90:23–32.

24. Guldbrand H, Dizdar B, Bunjaku B. et al. In type 2 diabetes, randomisation to advice to follow a low-carbohydrate diet transiently improves glycaemic control compared with advice to follow a low-fat diet producing a similar weight loss. *Diabetologia* 2012;55:2118–2127.

25. Brehm BJ, Seeley RJ, Daniels SR, D'Alessio DA. A randomized trial comparing a very low carbohydrate diet and a calorie-restricted low fat diet on body weight and cardio-vascular risk factors in healthy women. *J Clin Endocrinol Metab* 2003;88:1617–1623.

26. Nickols-Richardson SM, Coleman MM, Volpe JM, Hosig KW. Perceived hunger is lower and weight loss is greater in overweight premenopausal women consuming a low-carbohydrate/high-protein vs high-carbohydrate/low-fat diet. *J Am Diet Assoc* 2005;105:1433–1437.

27. McClernon FJ, Yancy WS Jr, Eberstein JA. et al. The effects of a low-carbohydrate ketogenic diet and a low-fat diet on mood, hunger, and other self-reported symptoms. *Obesity*. 2007 Jan;15(1):182–187.

28. Nouvenne A, Ticinesi A, Morellli I. et al. Fad diets and their effect on urinary stone formation. *Transl Androl Urol* 2014;3(3):303–312.

29. Iguchi M, Umekawa T, Takamura C. et al. Glucose metabolism in renal stone patients. *Urol Int*. 1993;51(4):185–90.

30. Nguyen NU, Dumoulin G, Henriet MT. et al. Carbohydrate metabolism and urinary excretion of calcium and oxalate after ingestion of polyol sweeteners. *J Clin Endocrinol Metab*. 1993;77(2):388–392.

31. Curhan GC, Willett WC, Speizer FE. et al. Comparison of dietary calcium with supple-mental calcium and other nutrients as factors affecting the risk for kidney stones in women. *An Int Med* 1997;126(7):497–504.

32. Holl MG, Allen LH. Sucrose ingestion, insulin response and mineral metabolism in humans. *J Nutr* 1987;117:1229–1233.

33. Reddy ST, Wang CY, Sakhaee K. et al. Effect of low-carbohydrate high-protein diets on acid-base balance, stone-forming propensity, and calcium metabolism. *Am J Kidney Dis*. 2002 Aug;40(2):265–274.

34. Von Geijer L, Ekelund M. Ketoacidosis associated with low-carbohydrate diet in a non-diabetic lactating woman: A case report. *J Med Case Rep* 2015;9:224.

2 DASH Diet

Thomas J. Moore, Megan Murphy,
and Lin Pao-Hwa

CONTENTS

OVERVIEW

The DASH (Dietary Approaches to Stop Hypertension) diet was developed and tested to help slow the rising incidence of hypertension in the United States. The original trial was a controlled feeding study, funded by the National Heart, Lung, and Blood Institute, and was conducted from 1993 to 1996 in five centers across the United States located in Boston, Massachusetts, Durham, North Carolina, Baltimore, Maryland, Baton Rouge, Louisiana, and Portland, Oregon.

This was a randomized control trial that included 459 study participants (average age 44 years; 49% women) with either prehypertension or stage 1 hypertension (overall eligible blood pressure range was 80–95 mm Hg diastolic and <160 mm Hg systolic). After eating a typical American (control) diet for three weeks, participants were randomly assigned to one of three diets for an eight-week period; the typical American diet (control diet), the typical American diet with added fruits and vegetables, or the DASH Diet. All three diets contained the same amount of sodium. Each participant visited the study location once per day (Monday through Friday) to consume the main meal for the day and took the rest of his or her food to eat at home. Adherence was monitored by directly observing the participants eating their main meal of the day and verified via periodic analysis of urinary electrolytes. Caloric intake was adjusted throughout the study to ensure baseline weights were maintained.

After two weeks, study participants eating the DASH Diet lowered their blood pressure by an average of 5.5/3 mm Hg and this reduction remained through the eight-week intervention. For those with a blood pressure greater than or equal to 140/90 mm Hg at baseline and who were also assigned to the DASH Diet group, blood pressure was lowered by an average of 11.4/5.5 mm Hg. In addition to blood pressure reduction, the DASH Diet also lowered total cholesterol an average of 14 mg/dL.[1]

Subsequent studies have shown that the DASH Diet also promotes weight loss and has beneficial effects on several other health outcomes (see *Current Research* section).

WHAT IS THE DASH DIET?

The DASH Diet emphasizes fruits, vegetables, whole grains, and low-fat dairy, and is reduced in meats, saturated fats, and sweets. The DASH Diet was originally designed with the goal of reaching a certain intake level of selected nutrients that were hypothesized to benefit blood pressure control. These nutrients include protein, fiber, potassium, magnesium, and calcium. After the DASH Diet was proven to be very effective in blood pressure reduction, it was translated and introduced to the public as a dietary pattern characterized by eight food groups: Fruits, Vegetables, Grains, Dairy, Meats, Nuts/Seeds/Legumes, Added Fats, and Sweets.

HOW TO FOLLOW THE DASH DIET

Getting started requires three steps:

1. Calculate daily calorie needs. There are many online sites and apps that offer calorie calculators (e.g., MyFitnessPal, 360HealthWatch, dashforhealth.com, and the DASH Food Tracker app). These sites will calculate how many calories one needs to maintain current weight. If weight loss is desired, subtract 500 calories from the calories needed for weight maintenance.
2. Determine the number of daily servings of each DASH food group (Table 2.1) based on the calorie need calculated in Step 1 above.
3. Learn what is a DASH "serving" in each food group:

Fruits

- One medium piece of fruit (about the size of a tennis ball)
- 1/2 of a large piece of fruit (grapefruit, 7-inch banana)

TABLE 2.1
DASH Servings Goals for a Range of Daily Calorie Intakes

Calorie Target	Grains	Fruits	Vegetables	Dairy	Meats	Nuts/Seeds/ Legumes	Added Fats	Sweets
1200	5	3	4	2	1.5	0.25	0.5	0.5
1400	5	4	4	2	1.5	0.25	0.5	0.5
1600	6	4	4	2	1.5	0.25	1	0.5
1800	6.5	4	4	2.5	1.5	0.5	1.5	0.5
2000	7	4	4	2.5	1.5	0.5	2	0.5
2200	8	4	5	3	2	0.5	2.5	1
2400	9	5	5	3	2	0.5	3	1
2600	10	5	5	3	2.5	1	3	1.5
2800	11	6	6	3.5	2.5	1	4	2

- 6 ounces (oz.) of 100% fruit juice (limit to one serving per day)
- 1/2 cup chopped fruit or berries
- 1/4 cup dried fruit

Vegetables

- 1 cup of uncooked leafy vegetables
- 1/2 cup cooked vegetables
- 1/2 cup non-leafy vegetables (peppers, cucumber, broccoli, corn, etc.)
- 6 oz. 100% vegetable juice
- 1/2 cup tomato sauce or other stewed vegetables
- 1/2 medium potato (about the size of a computer mouse)

Dairy

- 8 oz. of low-fat milk, yogurt, or cottage cheese
- 1 1/2 oz. of low-fat cheese
- 4 oz. low-fat frozen yogurt or ice cream (limit to one serving per day)

Grains (select at least half as whole grains)

- 1 oz. of bread, cereal, crackers, pretzels, etc.
- 1/2 cup cooked pasta, rice, cereal (like oatmeal or cream of wheat)

Meat (this includes meat, fish, poultry, and eggs)

- 3 oz. cooked meat, fish, poultry
- 3 eggs
- 6 egg whites

Meat alternatives

- 3 oz. seitan
- 9 oz. tofu
- 4 oz. tempeh
- 1/2 cup texturized vegetable protein

Nuts, seeds, and legumes

- 1/3 cup nuts
- 1/2 cup cooked beans/legumes
- 2 tablespoons of seeds

Added fats

- 1 teaspoon of butter, margarine, or oil
- 1 tablespoon of regular salad dressing, mayonnaise, cream cheese, sour cream, and dairy cream
- 2 tablespoons of low fat varieties of salad dressing and mayonnaise

Sweets

- 6 oz. sugar-sweetened beverages such as soft drinks, juice cocktails, and punches
- 1 tablespoon sugar, syrup, jelly, or jam
- 1 ounce candy (hard candies, gummy, or sours) or chocolate

Sodium

While technically not a food group, sodium is worth addressing here. In the original DASH Trial, we demonstrated that the DASH Diet lowered blood pressure when participants were consuming a diet with moderate sodium reduction (3000 mg/d). But in the DASH-Sodium Trial, we demonstrated that the DASH Diet lowered blood pressure even more effectively when combined with a greater reduction in sodium intake.[2] For participants with high blood pressure or prehypertension, we recommend that they limit their sodium intake to 1500 mg/day by avoiding sodium-rich foods and reducing added salt during cooking and at the table.

HOW THE DIET WORKS

Although the DASH Diet has been shown to have several health benefits, the primary reason for designing the DASH Diet was to find an eating pattern that would lower blood pressure even without weight loss or sodium reduction. So we will limit our discussion of how the DASH Diet works to what is known about its effect on blood pressure.

This question, how does it work, can be interpreted in two ways. One could be asking what component (or components) of the DASH Diet exerts its blood pressure lowering effect. Alternatively, one could be asking through what mechanism of action does the DASH Diet work. Although these are probably the most commonly asked questions about the DASH Diet, we do not have definitive answers to either one. However, past research does raise some possibilities that are worth exploring.

WHAT COMPONENT(S) OF THE DASH DIET LOWER BLOOD PRESSURE (BP)?

Many previous studies have evaluated the blood pressure effects of individual micro and macronutrients as well as specific nutrients in combination. As mentioned earlier, in designing the DASH Diet, we tried to incorporate the dietary components that these

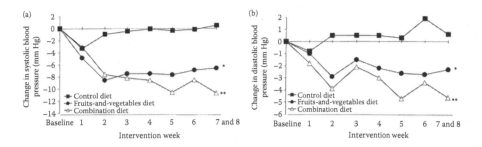

FIGURE 2.1 Systolic (a) and diastolic (b) blood pressure responses in the 133 hypertensive participants in the DASH Trial. The DASH Diet group is identified here as "Combination Diet."[8]

previous studies had suggested might lower blood pressure. These included increased consumption of potassium,[3] magnesium,[4] and calcium[5] as well as fiber[6] and protein.[7] The design of the DASH Trial does not allow an evaluation of these components individually because they were always delivered as whole foods, with their complex mixture of other macro and micronutrients. However, the DASH Trial did test three different diets: a control diet (comparable to the typical American diet), a diet rich in fruits and vegetables but comparable to the control diet in its content of meat, grains, and dairy foods (the F/V diet), and the DASH Diet. By comparing the macronutrient and micronutrient contents of these three diets versus their blood pressure effect, we can draw some inferences about which dietary components influenced blood pressure.

The F/V diet lowered blood pressure approximately half as much as the DASH Diet. Looking just at the 133 hypertensive participants studied in the DASH Trial,[8] the F/V diet (compared to the control diet) was associated with a blood pressure change of −7.2/−2.8 mm Hg (systolic/diastolic) while the DASH Diet was associated with a blood pressure change of −11.4/−5.5 mm Hg (Figure 2.1). So comparing the control diet and the F/V diet could identify components that caused a partial blood pressure effect. Then the differences between the F/V and DASH Diets would indicate the components that lead to the remaining blood pressure effect.

Table 2.2 shows the number of daily servings in each of the eight DASH food groups, and the macronutrient and micronutrient contents for the three diets. The italics format identifies how diet components differ among the three diets. These differences are summarized in Table 2.3.

The components in the left column of Table 2.3 likely contribute to a portion of the DASH BP effect. Adding the characteristics in the right column results in the full DASH effect.

In some instances, increased intake of specific micro or macronutrients is tied to increased servings of specific food groups. For example, increased potassium and fiber intake are related especially to increased servings of fruits and vegetables and increased calcium intake is related to increased servings of dairy food.

Further, food groups like red meat, whole fat dairy, and added animal fats were reduced in order to reduce saturated fat intake. Sugar-sweetened foods and beverages were also reduced mainly because there is just not much room for calorie-dense and nutrient-poor foods in the DASH Diet. Is it possible that certain foods and nutrients

TABLE 2.2
Daily Food Group Servings, Macronutrients (as % of Daily Calories), and Micronutrients in the Three Diets Tested in DASH Trial (2100 cal/day Level)[1]

	Control	F/V	DASH
Daily Servings			
Fruits	1.6	5.2	5.2
Vegetables	2	3.3	4.4
Grains	8.2	6.9	7.5
Dairy	0.5	0.3	2.7
Meat	2.5	2.5	1.6
Nuts/Seeds/Legumes	0	0.6	0.7
Fats	5.8	5.3	2.5
Sweets	4.1	1.4	0.7
Macronutrients %			
Carbohydrate	48	48	55
Total fat	37	37	27
Saturated fat	16	16	6
Monounsaturated fat	13	13	13
Polyunsaturated fat	8	8	8
Protein	15	15	18
Fiber (g/day)	9	31	31
Micronutrients			
Sodium (mg)	3000	3000	3000
Potassium (mg)	1700	4700	4700
Magnesium (mg)	165	500	500
Calcium (mg)	450	450	1240

Source: Appel, LJ et al. *N Engl J Med* 1997;336:1117–24.

Note: Components in italics are those where the F/V and the DASH Diet are the same but both are different from the control diet (partial blood pressure effect). Components in bold italics are those where the DASH Diet differs from both F/V and control diets (remaining blood pressure effect).

raise blood pressure? Reducing those foods might then contribute to DASH's blood pressure lowering effect.

Reducing red meat: In designing the DASH Diet, consumption of red meat was reduced largely to reduce saturated fat intake. The accompanying decrease in total protein intake was offset by an increase in protein from plant sources. Studies of the blood pressure effect of protein intake have documented that increased protein intake lowers blood pressure and that plant protein has more blood pressure effect than animal protein. We know of no evidence that red meat consumption directly raises blood pressure. But it is possible that

---

TABLE 2.3

Food Group and Nutrient Comparison of the Three Diets

F/V and DASH differ from control diet	DASH differs from F/V diet
↑ Fruit servings	↑ Dairy servings
↑ Vegetable servings	↓ Meat/fish/poultry servings
↑ Nuts/legumes servings	↓ Fat servings
↓ Sweets servings	
↑ Fiber	↑ Carbohydrate
↑ Potassium	↓ Saturated fat
↑ Magnesium	↑ Protein
	↑ Calcium

---

replacing red meat in DASH with protein from plant sources contributed to the DASH blood pressure effect.[9]

Reducing saturated fat: Published studies have shown a modest blood pressure lowering effect from increased consumption of monounsaturated fats.[10,11] But intake of monounsaturated fats was similar in all three diets tested in the DASH Trial (13% of total calories). There is no evidence that saturated fat intake has a direct blood pressure effect.

Reducing sugar-sweetened foods and beverages: In the DASH Diet, sugar consumption is significantly lower than in the average American diet. But the DASH Diet is not a low carbohydrate diet. In fact, its carbohydrate content is higher than the average American diet. But this increase in carbohydrate intake comes mainly from complex carbohydrates in fruits, vegetables, and whole grain products—not from simple sugars. Many previous studies have examined the effect of carbohydrate on blood pressure, including studies of total carbohydrate, high versus low-glycemic index, and various sugars. Cross-sectional analysis of the 2003–2006 NHANES cohort showed a direct association between fructose intake and blood pressure in adults,[12] but the results of other trials of simple sugar intake are inconclusive. Beyond studies of simple sugar intake, studies of various carbohydrates are also inconclusive. Perhaps most relevant to our assessment of the DASH Diet, Sacks and colleagues[13] conducted a cross-over controlled feeding study that assessed four diets, each for five weeks. Each diet was designed on the platform of the DASH Diet: low carb/low glycemic index; low carb/high glycemic index; high carb/low glycemic index; and high carb/high glycemic index. They found no difference in the blood pressure lowering effect of these four diets, despite their significant differences in both the amount and type of carbohydrate. All four diets lowered systolic pressure by 7–9 mm Hg and diastolic by 4–6 mm Hg.

Based on the evidence from previous studies, it seems unlikely that reducing red meat, saturated fat or simple sugar intake in the DASH Diet all play a significant role in the diet's overall blood pressure effect. However, each of these foods and nutrient factors may have contributed in part to the total blood pressure effect.

What Is the Mechanism of the DASH Diet's Blood Pressure Effect?

A number of studies have examined the mechanism by which the DASH Diet lowers blood pressure. Blood pressure is controlled by multiple systems, including the sympathetic nervous system, circulating factors like renin-angiotensin, and factors acting directly in resistance vessels such as nitric oxide, endothelin, and locally-produced angiotensin. In addition, there are different sensitivities to these factors in different individuals. Finally, any perturbation in blood pressure can evoke compensatory actions in these regulatory systems. This complexity makes understanding the mechanism of any blood pressure lowering intervention, including the DASH Diet, difficult to determine. However, previous studies have raised some possible mechanisms.

Svetkey and colleagues examined genetic polymorphisms in the angiotensinogen gene in participants who participated in the DASH Trial.[14] They found that one polymorphism, an arginine substitution for guanine in the −6 position, was associated with a greater blood pressure response to both the DASH and F/V diets. It has been speculated that this polymorphism may increase angiotensinogen levels and thereby the activity of the renin-angiotensin system (RAS). The greater blood pressure response in participants with this genetic pattern suggests that these diets may work through blockade or interruption of the RAS.

Studies have suggested that levels of plasma renin activity (PRA) increase in participants fed the DASH Diet.[15,16] Increased potassium intake can increase PRA levels, so this increase may simply be due to greater potassium intake. But natriuresis and even mild volume depletion can also increase PRA levels. Some have suggested that the DASH Diet causes sodium excretion and this results in its blood pressure lowering action.[15,17] But to date, no study has measured daily sodium excretion in the first days of consuming the DASH Diet to determine whether there is a natriuresis beyond that seen with a control diet.

The adrenergic nervous system has also been implicated. Urinary catecholamines are not different on the DASH versus control diets. But Sun and colleagues have examined how polymorphisms of the beta-2 adrenergic receptor gene affect the blood pressure response to the DASH Diet.[18] This receptor causes vasodilation and release of renin. It has been shown that a specific polymorphism of this gene (the AA allele at the G46A site) results in a receptor with blunted responsiveness to beta-2 agonists. Sun and colleagues found this AA genotype in 16% of white participants in the DASH Trial and 27% of the African Americans. These participants with the AA genotype also had a greater systolic pressure response to the DASH Diet as well as a blunted increase in PRA. The authors hypothesize that the blunted responsiveness of the beta-2 adrenergic receptor in this AA subset results in a blunted RAS counterregulatory response to the DASH-induced BP lowering, resulting in a greater BP effect in these participants.

As a final example of the mechanistic studies that have been performed, Lin and colleagues fed a group of hypertensive participants either the DASH or control diet for two weeks and measured vascular responsiveness.[15] They found that participants fed the DASH Diet had significantly greater post-ischemic plasma nitrite levels than the control diet group. They also had a reduction in vascular stiffness, measured as reduced carotid/posterior tibial pulse wave velocity. These observations suggest that the DASH Diet may exert an action at the level of the endothelium, increasing nitric oxide availability and reducing vascular stiffness.

CURRENT RESEARCH

Since the original DASH Trial was published in 1997, a number of additional studies have further examined the effect of this diet on blood pressure as well as other health outcomes. These studies have confirmed the effect of the DASH Diet on blood pressure as well as improving outcomes for other cardiovascular diseases, diabetes, cancer, and all-cause mortality.

DASH DIET AND BLOOD PRESSURE

DASH DIET PLUS SODIUM REDUCTION

The original DASH research team performed a follow-up controlled feeding study, combining the DASH Diet and various levels of sodium intake, to test whether DASH combined with sodium reduction was more effective than either intervention alone (DASH-Sodium Trial[2]). They tested a control diet and the DASH Diet, each on three different levels of sodium intake: 150, 100, and 50 mEq per day for 2100 cal per day intake (respectively, 3450, 2300, and 1150 mg Na). They found that both the DASH Diet and sodium reduction lowered blood pressure significantly and that DASH plus sodium reduction was more effective than either intervention alone (see systolic blood pressure responses in Table 2.4).

DASH DIET PLUS ANTIHYPERTENSIVE MEDICATIONS

Conlin and colleagues performed a controlled feeding study with hypertensive participants. Half were given a control diet for eight weeks and half the DASH Diet. Within each diet, there was a four week, crossover treatment with placebo and the angiotensin receptor blocker, losartan (50 mg).[19] On the control diet, losartan lowered 24-hour systolic ambulatory blood pressure (ABP) by 6.7 mm Hg. The DASH Diet alone lowered systolic ABP by 5.3 mm Hg. Adding losartan to the DASH Diet lowered systolic ABP by an additional 11.7 mm Hg. The authors concluded that combining the DASH Diet with antihypertensive medications may lead to additional blood pressure lowering benefit. Although the DASH Diet did not change plasma renin activity overall, the enhanced response to losartan in the DASH Diet group

TABLE 2.4
Systolic Blood Pressure Effect of DASH Diet and Sodium Reduction[2]

	150 mEq Na	100 mEq Na	50 mEq Na
Control diet	Reference	−2.1 mm Hg	−6.7 mm Hg
DASH Diet	−5.9 mm Hg	−7.2 mm Hg	−8.9 mm Hg

might suggest that the DASH Diet may have activated the renin-angiotensin system (perhaps at the local, vascular level), sensitizing participants to angiotensin blockade.

DASH Diet in Free-Choice Setting

Both the DASH and the DASH-Sodium Trials were controlled feeding studies where all the foods were purchased and prepared for all the participants for the duration of the studies. This assures adherence to the intervention diets, but may give an exaggerated idea of what these diets could accomplish in a real-world setting where participants make their own food decisions and adherence would be less predictable. Blumenthal and colleagues tested the DASH Diet in a more real-world setting (the ENCORE study[20]). They randomly assigned 144 untreated hypertensive participants into three diet groups: a control diet group, a DASH Diet group, and a DASH Diet plus weight loss group. Participants followed their diet assignments for four months. The DASH Diet group had weekly sessions with the nutritionist to reinforce the diet. The DASH Diet plus weight loss group had additional weekly cognitive behavioral sessions and supervised exercise sessions 3 times per week involving 10 minutes of warm-up exercises, 30 minutes of biking and/or walking or jogging, and 5 minutes of cool-down exercises. At the end of four months, the control diet group showed a 3.8 mm Hg reduction in clinic-measured systolic pressure, compared to a reduction of 11.2 mm Hg in the DASH Diet group. The DASH Diet plus weight loss resulted in a 16.1 mm Hg reduction in systolic pressure.

Modifying the DASH Diet

In the original DASH Trial, we observed that the DASH Diet reduced total cholesterol (−13.7 mg/dL), low-density lipoprotein (LDL) cholesterol (10.7 mg/dL), and high-density lipoprotein (HDL) cholesterol (−3.7 mg/dL) compared to the control diet group. To test whether altering the composition of the DASH Diet could retain its blood pressure and LDL lowering effect but avoid the HDL lowering effect, Appel and colleagues conducted a trial that compared a DASH-like diet, a DASH-like diet with 10% more calories from protein (CHO content was reduced by 10%), and a DASH-like diet with 10% more calories from fat, predominantly monounsaturated fat (the OmniHeart Trial[11]). Both modified diets reduced blood pressure slightly more than the DASH-like diet. And the fat-enriched diet reduced HDL cholesterol less than both of the other diets. The authors concluded that modifying the macronutrient content of the DASH Diet might preserve its blood pressure benefit while offering more favorable lipid effects. However, it is relevant to note that the DASH-like diet studied in OmniHeart was different from the DASH Diet studied in the original DASH Trial. In OmniHeart, the DASH-like diet provided 3% fewer calories from protein and 3% more from carbohydrate. These changes may have blunted the blood pressure effect of the DASH-like diet while having an unknown effect on lipids.

Another study examined the DASH Diet with modified carbohydrate content. Sacks and colleagues conducted a feeding study of four diets, each based on the DASH Diet: low carb/low glycemic index; low carb/high glycemic index; high carb/ low glycemic index; and high carb/high glycemic index (the OmniCarb trial).[13] They found no difference in the blood pressure lowering effects of these four diets. They concluded that the amount or type of carbohydrate did not influence the blood pressure effect of the DASH Diet.

OTHER HEALTH EFFECTS OF THE DASH DIET

In addition to the direct intervention studies cited above, numerous observational studies have examined the effect of the DASH Diet on an array of health conditions. Typically, these studies have used a validated DASH Diet index to analyze the reported food intake of the study cohort and then related greater or less adherence to the DASH Diet versus a health outcome.

CARDIOVASCULAR DISEASE

A number of studies have been published on this topic. Salehi-Abargouei and colleagues published a systematic review and meta-analysis of this literature and included six observational studies that calculated DASH Diet adherence and cardiovascular outcomes in participants without pre-existing cardiovascular disease.[21] The cohorts in these studies included the Nurses' Health Study, the Women's Health Study, EPICOR, the Swedish Mammography cohort, the Cohort of Swedish Men, and the Iowa Women's Health Study. Three of these studies examined the relationship of the DASH Diet and coronary heart disease (CHD). The relative risk of CHD in the most DASH adherent group compared to the least adherent was 0.79 (in 144,337 participants). Three studies included data on stroke incidence. The relative risk of stroke in the highest versus lowest DASH adherence groups was 0.81 (150,191 participants). Finally, two studies examined congestive heart failure. The relative risk of developing heart failure in the highest versus lowest DASH adherent groups was 0.71 (74,966 participants).

CANCER

Jones-McLean and colleagues reported a significant inverse relationship between DASH Diet and colorectal cancer (CRC) in Canadian men (relative risk [RR] 0.67 in highest versus lowest DASH adherence groups).[22] Fung and colleagues also reported a significant inverse relationship between DASH eating score and CRC participant in the Nurses' Health Study and the Health Professionals Study (132,000 participants).[23] Comparing the top and bottom quintiles of the DASH scores, the pooled RR for CRC was 0.80. These investigators found no association with CRC and the diet score using the Alternative Mediterranean Diet Index. Vargas and colleagues examined the relationship between diet quality and CRC incidence in the Women's Health Initiative Observational Study (93,700 women; 12.4 years follow-up).[24] They analyzed diet quality with four diet index scoring systems, including the DASH index. They found adherence scores in the DASH Diet index and the Healthy Eating Index 2010 were associated with significant reduction in CRC incidence (RR = 0.78 and 0.73, respectively). The Alternative Healthy Eating Index and the Alternative Mediterranean Diet Index were not associated with lower CRC risk. Hirko and colleagues examined diet quality and breast cancer risk, according to the molecular subtype of the cancers in 100,643 women in the Nurses' Health Study.[25] They found a significant risk reduction in HER2 type breast cancer and DASH Diet adherence (HR 0.44 in highest versus lowest adherence quintiles). Neither the Alternative Healthy Eating Index nor the Alternative Mediterranean Diet Index showed any significant association with breast cancer risk in this study.

COGNITION

In a subset of the ENCORE study cohort reviewed above, Smith and colleagues performed a prospective intervention study of 124 hypertensive participants, assigning them to three study arms for four months: control diet, DASH Diet, and DASH Diet plus behavioral therapy and exercise for weight loss.[26] They administered a battery of neurocognitive tests at baseline and end of study. Compared to the control diet group, the DASH participants showed significant improvement in psychomotor speed and the DASH-weight loss group showed improvement in both psychomotor speed and executive function/learning. Wengreen and colleagues conducted a prospective observational cohort study of 3831 men and women >65 years old.[27] Cognitive function tests were administered 4 times over an 11 year period and diet quality was assessed using DASH Diet and Mediterranean Diet indices. Participants in the highest quintiles for both the DASH and Mediterranean eating patterns scored consistently higher on cognitive testing over the 11 years. Tangney and colleagues reported similar findings in 825 elderly participants in the Memory and Aging Project.[28] Participants with higher DASH or Mediterranean Diet scores showed slower rates of cognitive decline on serial cognitive testing over four years (Figure 2.2).

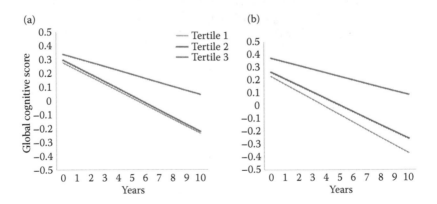

FIGURE 2.2   Cognitive change over time by DASH scores MedDietScores. Changes in global cognitive scores over time as a function of (a) DASH score tertiles and (b) MedDietScore tertiles. All mixed models included covariable adjustments by age, sex, education, energy, and late-life cognitive activities. Change rates in global congnitive scores of Memory and Aging Project participants were significantly associated in the highest tertiles of either score—DASH ($\beta = 0.022$, SEE = 0.011, $p = 0.04$) or MedDiet ($\beta = 0.034$, SEE = 0.012, $p = 0.003$)— but not for those DASH scores ($\beta = -0.001$, SEE = **0.010**, $p = 0.95$) or MedDietScores ($\beta = 0.01$, SEE = 0.011, $p = 0.37$) in the second tertiles. DASH = Dietary Approach to Stop Hypertension; MedDiet = Mediterranean Diet; MedDietScore = Mediterranean Diet score; SEE = standard error of estimate.

DIABETES

de Koning and colleagues examined the relationship between diet quality and the incidence of type 2 diabetes in 41,000 men in the Health Professionals Follow-up Study.[29] Diet quality was assessed every four years over 20 years of follow-up. Comparing the highest and lowest quintiles of DASH adherence, there was a 25% reduction in the incidence of type 2 diabetes. Similar reductions were seen when diet quality was scored with the Alternative Healthy Eating Index and the Alternative Mediterranean Diet Index. Another observational study also showed that adhering to the DASH dietary pattern reduced risk for diabetes among whites.[30]

WEIGHT LOSS

Hollis and colleagues[31] conducted a 6-month weight loss trial of lifestyle factors and diet. Overweight and obese participants (n = 1685) attended 20 weekly group sessions to encourage calorie restriction, moderate-intensity physical activity, and the DASH Diet. This was not a feeding study. Participants selected and consumed foods of their own choosing. After six months of this multifaceted intervention, mean weight loss was 5.8 kg. A follow-up trial (the Weight Loss Maintenance [WLM] Study[32]) examined how well the weight loss seen in the Hollis trial could be maintained. Participants who had lost at least 4 kg in the Hollis trial (average weight loss was 8.5 kg, n = 1032) were eligible for the WLM study. They were randomly assigned to one of three approaches to weight maintenance: monthly personal contact, unlimited access to an interactive technology-based intervention, or self-directed control. After 30 months, all three groups had regained some of their lost weight. The self-directed group regained 5.5 kg, 5.2 kg in the interactive technology group, and 4.0 kg in the personal-contact group. No group regained all the weight they had lost during the 6-month Hollis study.

To summarize, considerable research has shown an array of health benefits from consuming a DASH-type eating pattern in addition to its blood pressure benefit.

TYPICAL RESULTS

As described previously, many study participants in controlled feeding studies of the DASH eating pattern experienced significant lowering of blood pressure, improved lipids, and other markers of improved health.[1,2,15,19] Since all the foods were purchased and prepared for the participants in these studies, the adherence was very high (95%). However, when participants in subsequent studies were counseled how to choose foods and prepare foods themselves, the overall adherence decreased substantially.[33,34] In general, closer adherence to the DASH dietary pattern correlated with greater blood pressure and lipid improvement. A proportional relationship between adherence to the DASH dietary pattern and blood pressure outcome is also observed in observational studies where disease risk was assessed. A closer adherence to the DASH Diet is associated with a lower risk for cardiovascular disease and stroke. Although these results suggest that greater adherence to the DASH

Diet results in a greater health benefit, any adherence may also be beneficial and so should be encouraged. The DASH dietary pattern can be designed for any calorie level. Individuals can follow the DASH dietary pattern to fit their specific caloric needs including weight loss. And when individuals adopt the DASH eating pattern at a lower calorie level than they need to maintain current body weight, weight loss was observed.[32] Sample servings for various food group distributions are available for different calorie levels (see Table 2.1).

There are various factors that may affect how closely one adheres to the DASH eating pattern.

1. For most Americans, following the DASH eating pattern requires modification of several eating habits such as increasing intakes of fruits and vegetables and decreasing intake of sugar-sweetened foods. According to a recent dietary survey in the United States,[35] average intake of vegetables is about 1.4 serving/day, which is much lower than that recommended by DASH (4–5 servings/day). This is also true for other food groups where the current intake is quite different from the recommendation.[36] Thus, modifying the current eating behavior toward the DASH goal may require an amount of effort that many individuals may not be willing or ready to commit to. Identification of effective strategies to help individuals make the dietary changes and stay motivated to maintain the changes is an urgent need.

2. Food availability. Even though eating a healthy pattern like DASH does not need to cost more, it can be a real challenge for people living in low income neighborhoods to acquire healthy eating skills and practice healthy eating habits regularly. For example, availability of fruits and vegetables in such neighborhoods may be particularly limited, but this situation does not need to limit people from following the DASH Diet. On the one hand, more

---

TABLE 2.5

Comparison of Target DASH Nutrients to the Average American Intake in 2013–2014

Nutrients	2013–2014 Average American intake	DASH Diet Target
Total fat (%kcal)	34.7	27
Saturated fat (%kcal)	11.2	6
Protein (%kcal)	15.6	18
Fiber (g)	17.1	31
Potassium (mg)	2658	4700
Magnesium (mg)	305	500
Calcium (mg)	965	1240

Source: What We Eat in America, NHANES 2013–2014, individuals 2 years and over (excluding breast-fed children), day 1. Available: www.ars.usda.gov/nea/bhnrc/fsrg, accessed October 17, 2016.

education is needed to help individuals acquire healthy eating skills. On the other hand, systematic changes should be pursued to improve availability of healthy foods in low income neighborhoods.

3. Another challenge for many people is the lack of proper knowledge in selecting food choices that achieve the potassium and magnesium targets recommended by DASH.[37] Potassium content varies substantially from one food to another even within the same food group. For example, one cup of blueberries has 120 mg potassium while a cup of cantaloupe contains 495 mg. Choices of food items substantially impact the total nutrient intake. The original DASH study designed the DASH Diet based on a list of nutrients including potassium, calcium, magnesium, fats, and fiber. The target levels for these nutrients for a daily total caloric intake of 2100 cal is listed in Table 2.5. The dietary intakes of the average American based on the 2013–2014 NHANES survey are shown in the same table. There is a substantial difference between typical American intake and the DASH goals. In order to achieve the DASH target levels of these nutrients, conscientious effort is needed in making food choices.

PROS AND CONS OF FOLLOWING THE DASH DIET

Changing the way we eat is a challenge. We make decisions about what we eat based on numerous factors, including our preferences and our household, as well as simply what is convenient. As with all diets, including the DASH Diet, there are pros and cons to making healthy changes to the way we eat. Let's take a look at some of the benefits and challenges of eating the DASH way.

THE PROS: WELL-BALANCED, CUSTOMIZABLE, PROVEN, AND SAFE

The DASH Diet has many strengths but its greatest advantage over most other diets is its scientific credibility. Many scientific papers (some cited above) have reported its health benefits—from blood pressure and cholesterol reduction to cardiovascular disease to cognitive function.

All of the benefits of the DASH Diet can be enjoyed by just about anyone. This is because, while powerful, the DASH Diet is essentially very simple. It is a well-balanced way of eating made up of a diversity of foods. Anyone with access to a supermarket can follow the DASH Diet and it is customizable. For those with allergies, or strong food preferences, the DASH Diet can be followed by meeting the DASH recommended servings based on an individual's preference.

Choosing the right diet is a very personal decision. What works for one individual might not work for another. But the freedom to choose favorite foods within each food group allows individuals to select the foods they like—a definite advantage over more restricted diets. And the DASH Diet can prevent or treat a number of health problems.

The DASH Diet's safety and efficacy has made it one of the most heavily endorsed diets on the market today. It is recommended by the USDA, the JNC-7 High Blood Pressure Guidelines and the American Heart Association and has been ranked the #1

Overall Diet by *US News & World Report* every year since 2011. Clinicians recommend the DASH Diet to their patients for its health benefits, and the safety of the diet allows patients to follow it without the need for clinical supervision.

In addition to its effectiveness for certain disease states, the DASH Diet can be incorporated into a healthy weight loss plan. Finally, because it is a well-balanced, safe, and relatively easy eating pattern to follow, the DASH Diet can be recommended as the eating pattern for healthy people who just want to eat healthy and stay healthy. The DASH Diet is a pattern of eating that can be adopted *for life*.

THE CONS: PREFERENCE AND PLANNING

Anyone who has tried to change eating habits knows that it is a difficult task. Most are aware that eating more fruits and vegetables is a healthier option than swinging through the drive-thru on the way home from work. However, even setting simple dietary goals such as "I will eat more fruit this week," takes planning and effort. It takes *work and commitment* to adhere to a diet. When asked, dieters cite this reason as the number one challenge when starting the DASH Diet. The DASH Diet is a diet of whole foods enjoyed in their most natural form, and very little in the way of pre-packaged, processed foods. This means careful shopping and probably more time spent on food preparation compared to a diet of highly-processed, ready-to-eat food. There are exceptions such as yogurt and nuts that can be grabbed on the go, as well as shortcuts, like using frozen fruits and vegetables that do not spoil so they are more readily available, often cheaper, and quicker to prepare.

In addition to the work it takes to eat the DASH way, some people find that the diet's lower meat allowance is difficult. In the United States especially, typical diets are very meat-heavy. It can take a shift in thinking when first starting the DASH Diet, moving from meat as the centerpiece of the meal, shifting it to more of a side dish, then rounding out the meal with more whole grains and vegetables. Stir-fries and stews with plenty of vegetables are a great way to get around feeling meat-deprived.

Finally, a third barrier that is sometimes reported is the lack of restriction in the DASH Diet. The diet does not require participants to calorie count nor does it "forbid" certain food groups. Also, many of the foods promoted on the DASH Diet, such as unsaturated fats, nuts, and dried fruit and fruit juices are relatively high in calories. People interested in weight loss must consume these foods in moderation. Other weight loss diets avoid this issue by restricting entire food groups. In the DASH Diet, almost any food can be consumed *in moderation*.

IS THE DASH DIET RIGHT FOR YOUR PATIENT?

The DASH dietary pattern has been recommended by the American Dietary Guidelines since 2005 for individuals two years and older.[38] There are a few factors that any individual may want to consider as he/she starts to follow the DASH dietary pattern.

1. The DASH dietary pattern is safe for all individuals two years and older to follow with the exception of those with stage 4 or 5 chronic kidney disease or those prescribed by their health care providers to follow a reduced

potassium diet (<2000 mg). These individuals can still follow the DASH Diet as long as they avoid potassium-rich foods. Other features of the DASH eating pattern including lower sugar-sweetened foods, rich fiber, and magnesium are still beneficial for these individuals.

2. Following the DASH dietary pattern should ideally be a lifestyle decision and not an on/off type of short-term choice. Therefore, individuals must take time to move toward their DASH dietary goals (Table 2.1) and avoid the unrealistic expectation that one can achieve the DASH goals within a short time frame. Lasting change is the most powerful change.

3. Those who are interested in weight loss must be mindful of the total amount of food consumed. As discussed previously, the best strategy for weight loss is to subtract 500 calories from the calories needed to maintain current weight. Follow the three basic steps in the *How to Follow the DASH Diet* section above to get started on the DASH Diet. Make short-term and SMART (specific, measurable, actionable, realistic, and timed) goals and commit to them one by one. Utilize free online tools and phone apps such as the MyFitnessPal, 360HealthWatch, Dashforhealth.Com, and the DASH Diet Food Tracker app to help with monitoring caloric intake and keeping yourself accountable. Individuals have found these tools helpful with initiating dietary change and maintaining the changes long term.

4. Food intolerance or allergy. If individuals are intolerant or allergic to dairy products, it may be hard to adopt the DASH dietary pattern 100%. However, that does not mean it would not be worth the effort to adopt other aspects of this pattern. For some individuals, dairy intolerance may be relieved by taking lactase treated products or lactose free milk and dairy products, and some dairy products are naturally lower in lactose, such as yogurt, and may be better tolerated than milk.

5. Gluten sensitivity. Individuals with gluten sensitivity can choose grains without gluten and still follow the DASH pattern fully.

In conclusion, except for individuals with chronic kidney disease or those who should limit potassium intake, following the DASH dietary pattern is a lifestyle change that can benefit the vast majority of the population.

REFERENCES

1. Appel, LJ, Moore TJ, Obarzanek E. et al. A clinical trial of the effects of dietary patterns on blood pressure. *N Engl J Med* 1997;336:1117–24.
2. Sacks, FM, Svetkey, LP, Vollmer, WM. et al. Effects on blood pressure of reduced dietary sodium and the Dietary Approaches to Stop Hypertension (DASH) diet. DASH-Sodium Collaborative Research Group. *N Engl J Med* 2001;344:3–10.
3. Aburto, NJ, Hanson, S, Gutierrez, H. et al. Effect of increased potassium intake on cardiovascular risk factors and disease: Systematic review and meta-analyses. *BMJ* 2013;346:f1378.
4. Kass, L, Weekes, J, Carpenter, L. et al. Effect of magnesium supplementation on blood pressure: A meta-analysis. *Eur J Clin Nutr* 2012;66:411–8.

5. Van Mierlo, LA, Arends, LR, Streppel, MT. et al. Blood pressure response to calcium supplementation: A meta-analysis of randomized controlled trials. *J Hum Hypertens* 2006;20:571–80.

6. Hartley, L, May, MD, Loveman, E. et al. Dietary fibre for the primary prevention of cardiovascular disease. *Cochrane Database Syst Rev* 2016;(1):CD011472. doi: 10.1002/14651858.CD011472.pub2

7. Tielemans, SM, Altorf-van der Kuil, W, Engberink, MF. et al. Intake of total protein, plant protein and animal protein in relation to blood pressure: A meta-analysis of observational and intervention studies. *J Hum Hypertens* 2013;27:564–71.

8. Conlin, PR, Chow, D, Miller, ER 3rd. et al. The effect of dietary patterns on blood pressure control in hypertensive patients: Results from the Dietary Approaches to Stop Hypertension (DASH) trial. *Am J Hypertens* 2000;13:949–55.

9. Wang, YF, Yancy, WS, Yu, D. et al. The relationship between dietary protein intake and blood pressure: Results from the PREMIER study. *J Hum Hypertens* 2008;22:745–54.

10. Miura, K, Stamler, J, Brown IJ. et al. Relationship of dietary monounsaturated fatty acids to blood pressure: The international study of macro/micronutrients and blood pressure. *J Hypertens* 2013;31:1144–50.

11. Appel, LJ, Sacks, FM, Carey, VJ. et al. Effects of protein, monounsaturated fat, and carbohydrate intake on blood pressure and serum lipids: Results of the OmniHeart randomized trial. *J Amer Med Assoc* 2005;294:2455–64.

12. Jalal, DI, Smits, G, Johnson, RJ. et al. Increased fructose associates with elevated blood pressure. *J Am Soc Nephrol* 2010;21:1543–49.

13. Sacks, FM, Carey, VJ, Anderson, CA. et al. Effects of high vs low glycemic index of dietary carbohydrate on cardiovascular disease risk factors and insulin sensitivity: The OmniCarb randomized clinical trial. *JAMA* 2014;312:2531–41.

14. Svetkey, LP, Moore, TJ, Simons-Morton, DG. et al. Angiotensinogen genotype and blood pressure response in the Dietary Approaches to Stop Hypertension (DASH) study. *J Hypertens* 2001;19:1949–56.

15. Lin, PH, Allen, JD, Li, YJ. et al. Blood pressure-lowering mechanisms of the DASH dietary pattern. *J Nutr Metab* 2012; Article ID 2012:472396, doi: 10.11455/2012/472396.

16. Chen, Q, Turban, S, Millerm ER. et al. The effects of dietary patterns on plasma renin activity: Results from the Dietary Approaches to Stop Hypertension trial. *J Hum Hypertens* 2012;26:664–9.

17. Akita, S, Sacks, FM, Svetkey, LP. et al. Effects of the Dietary Approaches to Stop Hypertension (DASH) diet on the pressure-natriuresis relationship. *Hypertension* 2003;42:8–13.

18. Sun, B, Williams, JS, Svetkey, LP. et al. Beta2-adrenergic receptor genotype affects the renin-angiotensin-aldosterone system response to the Dietary Approaches to Stop Hypertension (DASH) dietary pattern. *Am J Clin Nutr* 2010;92:444–49.

19. Conlin, PR, Erlinger, TP, Bohannon, A. et al. The DASH diet enhances the blood pressure response to losartan in hypertensive patients. *Am J Hypertens* 2003;16:337–42.

20. Blumenthal, JA, Babyak, MA, Hinderliter, A. et al. Effects of the DASH diet alone and in combination with exercise and weight loss on blood pressure and cardiovascular biomarkers in men and women with high blood pressure: The ENCORE study. *Arch Intern Med* 2010;170:126–35.

21. Salehi-Abargouei, A, Maghsoudi, Z, Shirani, F, Azadbakht, L. Effects of Dietary Approaches to Stop Hypertension (DASH)-style diet on fatal or nonfatal cardiovascular diseases—incidence: A systematic review and meta-analysis on observational prospective studies. *Nutrition* 2013;29:611–8.

22. Jones-McLean, E, Hu, J, Greene-Finestone, LS. et al. A DASH dietary pattern and the risk of colorectal cancer in Canadian adults. *Health Promot Chronic Dis Prev Can* 2015;35:12–20.
23. Fung, TT, Hu, FB, Wu, K. et al. The Mediterranean and Dietary Approaches to Stop Hypertension (DASH) diets and colorectal cancer. *Am J Clin Nutr* 2010;92:1429–35.
24. Vargas, AJ, Neuhouser, ML, George, SM et al. Diet Quality and Colorectal Cancer Risk in the Women's Health Initiative Observational Study. *Am J Epidemiol* 2016;184:23–32.
25. Hirko, KA, Willett, WC, Hankinson, SE. et al. Healthy dietary patterns and risk of breast cancer by molecular subtype. *Breast Cancer Res Treat* 2016;155:579–88.
26. Smith, PJ, Blumenthal, JA, Babyak, MA. et al. Effects of the dietary approaches to stop hypertension diet, exercise, and caloric restriction on neurocognition in overweight adults with high blood pressure. *Hypertension* 2010;55:1331–8.
27. Wengreen, H, Munger, RG, Cutler, A. et al. Prospective study of Dietary Approaches to Stop Hypertension- and Mediterranean-style dietary patterns and age-related cognitive change: The Cache County Study on Memory, Health and Aging. *Am J Clin Nutr* 2013;98:1263–71.
28. Tangney, CC, Li, H, Wang, Y. et al. Relation of DASH- and Mediterranean-like dietary patterns to cognitive decline in older persons. *Neurology* 2014;83:1410–6.
29. de Koning, L, Chiuve, SE, Fung, TT. et al. Diet-quality scores and the risk of type 2 diabetes in men. *Diabetes Care* 2011;34:1150–6.
30. Liese, AD, Nichols, M, Sun, X. et al. Adherence to the DASH Diet is inversely associated with incidence of type 2 diabetes: The insulin resistance atherosclerosis study. *Diabetes Care* 2009;32:1434–6.
31. Hollis, JF, Gulliion, CM, Stevens, VJ. et al. Weight loss during the intensive intervention phase of the weight-loss maintenance trial. *Am J Prev Med* 2008;35:118–26.
32. Svetkey, LP, Stevens, VJ, Brantley, PJ. et al. Comparison of strategies for sustaining weight loss: The weight loss maintenance randomized controlled trial. *J Amer Med Assoc* 2008;299: 1139–48.
33. Svetkey, LP, Pollak, KI, Yancy, WS, Jr. et al. Hypertension improvement project: Randomized trial of quality improvement for physicians and lifestyle modification for patients. *Hypertension* 2009;54:1226–33.
34. Appel, LJ, Champagne, CM, Harsha, DW et al. Effects of comprehensive lifestyle modification on blood pressure control: Main results of the PREMIER clinical trial. *J Amer Med Assoc* 2003;289:2083–93.
35. National Cancer Institute. 2016. Usual Dietary Intakes: Food Intakes, U.S. Population, 2007-10. Epidemiology and Genomics Research Program website. Available at https://epi.grants.cancer.gov/diet/usualintakes/pop/2007-10/ (accessed February 1, 2017).
36. Rehm, CD, Penalvo, JL, Afshin, A. et al. Dietary intake among US adults, 1999-2012. *J Amer Med Assoc* 2016;315:2542–53.
37. Lin, PH, Appel, LJ, Funk, K. et al. The PREMIER intervention helps participants follow the Dietary Approaches to Stop Hypertension dietary pattern and the current Dietary Reference Intakes recommendations. *J Amer Dietetic Assoc* 2007;107:1541–51.
38. U.S. Department of Health and Human Services and U.S. Department of Agriculture. *2015–2020 Dietary Guidelines for Americans.* 8th edition. December 2015. Available at http://health.gov/dietaryguidelines/2015/guidelines/ (accessed February 1, 2017).

3 iDiet

Susan B. Roberts, Amy Krauss,
Madeleine M. Gamache, and Sai Krupa Das

CONTENTS

OVERVIEW

The high national prevalence of obesity and overweight is one of the major public health challenges of our time. Excess body weight not only increases the risk of chronic diseases and cognitive decline throughout adult life, but also dramatically increases health care costs.[1] Behavioral weight loss programs are recommended by expert committees for weight loss and prevention of weight regain,[2,3] and 5%–10% weight loss is a clinical benchmark recognized to provide important health benefits including decreased risk of diabetes and reduction in cardiometabolic risk factors.[2] However, scalable behavioral programs typically result in a mean weight loss of only 1%–5% in completing participants[4–10] and weight regain is common, which means that less than half of participants achieve clinically impactful weight loss.

The iDiet is a new healthy eating and weight loss program for sustainable weight loss built on novel principles. The program is disseminated both as a self-help book (*The "I" Diet* by Susan B. Roberts and Betty Kelly Sargent, Workman Publishing, 2010) and as a behavioral program (www.theidiet.com). The iDiet is a menu-based eating plan with behavioral support for the core goals of the program, which are hunger suppression and changing food preferences to decrease food cravings. These two factors have not been prioritized in conventional behavioral programs, yet have been shown to be associated with improved long-term weight control.[11,12] Hunger is thought to be important because it is known to be a key driver of food intake during attempts to lose weight. The 1944 Minnesota Starvation Study, as an extreme example, demonstrated that prolonged food deprivation caused severe hunger and resulted in numerous problems, including increases in hysteria, depression, and severe anxiety.[13] Even relatively short term periods of fasting that increase hunger can alter eating behavior patterns; for example, research studies have shown that fasted individuals select higher calorie starchy foods over nutrient-dense vegetables compared to non-fasted controls.[14]

The iDiet has been tested for effectiveness in a 12-month randomized controlled trial that compared iDiet implemented as an intensive behavioral program to a waitlisted control in four Boston, Massachusetts worksites. A series of four papers[11,12,15,16] were published on the trial results, with the primary outcome being 8% weight loss over six months (Figure 3.1), which is a higher mean value than reports for other scalable programs. In addition, there was no significant weight regain after 12 months. There were also significant improvements in blood pressure, total and low-density lipoprotein (LDL) cholesterol, and fasting blood glucose, together with reductions in self-reported food cravings and hunger. Moreover, and unusually for a behavioral weight loss program, the successful results were obtained among participants from a broad range of socioeconomic circumstances and racial and ethnic groups.

A commercial version of the program has been established and a recent analysis of program data reported a mean weight loss in completing enrollees of 6.4% over 11 weeks in 2013, rising to 7.2% in 2014, and 8.6% in 2015 (Figure 3.2),[1] with no

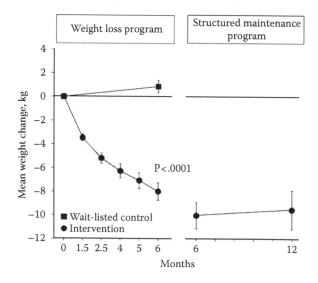

FIGURE 3.1 Change in weight for control and intervention enrollees during a 6-month iDiet weight loss program and a 6-month structured weight maintenance program. (Adapted from Salinardi TC. et al. *American Journal of Clinical Nutrition* 2013;97(4):667–76.)

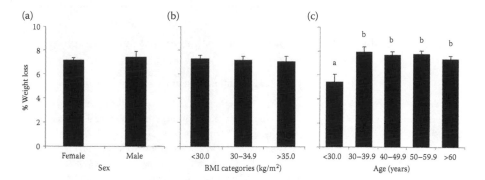

FIGURE 3.2 Percent weight loss in participants completing an 11-week iDiet program. Presented data are from Analysis of Covariance (ANCOVA) models adjusted for baseline weight, age category, class type, program delivery, start year and month. Letters a, b denotes levels with significant differences at the 0.05 level, adjusted using Turkey's HSD. (Adapted from Das SK. et al. *Obesity* 2017; 25(6):1033–41.)

difference in percent weight loss between programs delivered by videoconference and programs delivered in person. In addition, weight loss in participants enrolling in a second 11-week program, for a combined program duration of 22 weeks, was 13.5%.[1] By comparison, the original Diabetes Prevention Program, which is considered a model for intensive behavioral programs, achieved 7% mean weight loss over 6 months,[17] and commercial weight loss programs such as Weight Watchers typically achieve 4%–5% weight loss in completing participants.[18,19]

HOW DOES THE iDIET PROGRAM COMPARE TO CONVENTIONAL BEHAVIORAL PROGRAMS?

The iDiet has several features in common with conventional behavioral programs such as the Diabetes Prevention Program, and also some specific differences, as summarized in Table 3.1. Common features include acknowledging the importance of calories consumed versus calories expended, a goal of 1–2 lb. per week of weight loss, and implementation features including education on the importance of planning, use of problem solving strategies, and how to build social support.[20–34] Specific differences between iDiet and the Diabetes Prevention Program are related to underlying conceptual differences. Conventional behavioral programs are typically based on goal-setting theory[35] and apply standard behavioral skills training, such as creating behavioral targets, self-monitoring, and problem solving around stimulus control, which are features that are no longer identified with one specific health behavior model.[36] In contrast, iDiet is based on Social Cognitive Theory (SCT),[37] including the usual application of SCT principles seen in Cognitive-Behavior Therapy (CBT).[38] SCT explains behavior change in terms of reciprocal determinism between the individual's behavior, personal factors, and the environment, and also acknowledges both the importance of observational learning and the centrality of raising self-efficacy for specific behavior changes through incremental mastery exercises.[37] SCT additionally recognizes that the reciprocal relationship between self, behavior, and environment provides opportunities for

TABLE 3.1

Comparison of the iDiet with conventional behavioral programs such as the Diabetes Prevention Program

	Diabetes Prevention Program	iDiet
Common features of the Diabetes Prevention Program and iDiet	• *Goals*: Weight loss goal (1–2 lb/week), dietary energy reduction (500–1000 kcal/week) consumed in regular meals and snacks, activity goal (150 minutes/week). • *Group structure*: Weekly 1 hour group classes initially, declining to monthly over time with additional booster sessions. Classes involve check in, educational unit to support intervention goals, and time for questions and answers. Individual check in with group leader at or between meetings. • *Behavioral skills training*: Self-monitoring weight, food, and activity, use of problem solving to achieve intervention goals via stimulus control and relapse prevention, social support. • *Provided materials*: menu examples and recipes supporting dietary goals, book(s) and study handouts to support study adherence, log for self-monitoring weight.	
Different dietary composition goals and implementation path	• *Goals*: low calorie, low energy density, low fat. • *Core strategy*: daily self-monitoring for calories and fat. • *Additional*: general healthy food guidelines (e.g., MyPlate), with optional menus and recipes.	• *Goals*: low calorie, high fiber (>40 g/d), moderately high protein (26% energy), low glycemic load (48% energy with low glycemic index carbs). • *Core strategy*: use of provided calorie-controlled menus and recipes. • *Additional*: general portion guidelines and self-monitoring for portion sizes.
Different behavioral strategies	• *Core strategies*: exercise demonstrations with exercise logs. • *Additional*: stress management; mindful eating.	• *Core strategies*: hunger suppression and craving reduction via adherence to specific provided menus and cognitive restructuring exercises. • *Additional*: optional portion size monitoring, raising self-efficacy.

using multiple avenues to create behavior change. The theory recognizes there will be periods of variable adherence, lapse, and relapse in any behavior change, all of which need to be addressed for long-term success. CBT focuses on factors such as the learning and unlearning of individual behaviors through cognitive restructuring, and these factors are central to the implementation of iDiet. The justifications for specific differences of iDiet are given in the following paragraphs.

Hunger Suppression and Dietary Composition

The iDiet prioritizes hunger suppression to a greater degree than other conventional behavioral programs, which alternatively place more emphasis on other factors potentially influencing energy balance such as physical activity and mindful eating. iDiet concentrates specifically on meal-to-meal hunger control on the grounds that hunger makes it both more difficult to be adherent to a calorie-reduced eating program and harder to modify other factors that impact adherence, such as planning ahead or food preparation. The prioritization of hunger is achieved in two ways: specific dietary composition targets for routine use, and the use of low-calorie hunger-suppressing "free foods" to manage hunger acutely.

Concerning the specific dietary composition targets of iDiet, food plans provide $\geq$40 g/day dietary fiber, and an average of 26% energy from protein and 48% from low glycemic index (GI) carbohydrates,[39] and are also relatively low in energy density.[40] These dietary recommendations are consistent with the Acceptable Macronutrient Distribution Ranges of the Dietary Reference Intakes,[41] except for dietary fiber, which is higher and similar to amounts reported to lower cardiometabolic risk factors.[42] The specific targets are derived from short-term studies of dietary composition and hunger, which typically report high dietary fiber, high protein, low energy density, and low GI carbohydrates, all of which have acute beneficial effects on hunger and/or satiety and short-term advantages for reducing energy intake.[43-50] In contrast, most long-term dietary trials have found no significant effects of these dietary parameters on weight loss,[19,51-53] but this may have been partly due to a lack of power in the individual studies. One meta-analysis[54] identified several studies examining the effects of the GI on weight loss over a period of five weeks to six months, and while there was no significant effect in the individual studies, the meta-analysis showed significantly greater weight loss in the low compared to high GI dietary groups (mean difference 1.1 kg, $p < 0.05$).

It is also important to note that the four dietary targets of iDiet are implemented *concurrently*. Other behavioral programs typically recommend focusing on calories, or on calories combined with a single dietary target such as dietary fat or energy density.[55] However, it is known that there are multiple afferent signals of energy balance that are differentially influenced by different dietary factors,[56] therefore, an additive impact of some or all of these multiple signaling pathways on energy balance is plausible.[57] In addition, there is a growing literature indicating differential individual responsiveness to different dietary composition factors. For example, our group and others have shown that an individual's insulin secretion in response to a standard oral glucose tolerance predicts how much weight is lost on high versus low glycemic load diets, with individuals having a high insulin secretion losing more weight when randomized to a low glycemic load diet compared to a high glycemic load diet.[58,59] The postulated effect in this case is that both circulating insulin and glucose are signals of body energy status,[56] and a low GI diet will counterbalance a high inherent insulin secretion. When multiple dietary targets are combined in one "additive" dietary prescription, the net synergistic effect may therefore be that a greater percentage of individuals are able to benefit due to there being at least one prescriptive factor that synergizes with their individual metabolic profile.

FOOD PREFERENCES AND CRAVING REDUCTION

In addition to standard behavioral topics, iDiet includes additional topics specific to supporting adherence to the program's novel goals for hunger reduction and retraining food preferences to reduce food cravings. These include menu repetition (to support habit formation), the use of "free foods" (specific listed foods with few calories that can be eaten *ad libitum*) for acute hunger relief, and cognitive restructuring exercise to help change food preferences.

PRACTICAL IMPLEMENTATION STRATEGIES

Practical implementation of iDiet involves use of provided self-selection menus and recipes that embed the nutritional and behavioral prescriptions of the intervention for at least two weeks and ideally longer, because the multiple goals of iDiet require prescriptive dietary and eating patterns that may enhance the ability of participants to be adherent.[60-62] This approach contrasts with programs such as the Diabetes Prevention Program, which encourage unrestricted self-selection of healthy food choices and food logging combined with general advice on calorie goals and the importance of low fat/low energy density food selections to achieve a calorie reduction. The provided menus and recipes in iDiet include foods with familiar tastes despite the different macronutrient composition, including hamburgers, lasagna, "fried" chicken, pizza, burritos, and desserts such as ice cream sundaes and chocolate pudding.

EXERCISE

Unlike standard behavioral programs, iDiet does not recommend increasing exercise in the beginning of the program but instead encourages exercise after weight loss is established. This difference is partly because exercise interventions have been shown to have only a limited effect on weight loss,[63] therefore, exercise is recommended for general health rather than weight loss *per se*. In addition, the cognitive burden and time requirement of performing additional exercise has the potential to reduce a subject's ability to be broadly adherent to the dietary prescription. Exercise goals are therefore phased in after dietary changes are established.

HOW TO FOLLOW THE iDIET PROGRAM

There are several different ways to follow the iDiet program. One is to independently use the menus, recipes, and behavioral strategies outlined in *The "I" Diet* book.[64] Patients can alternatively join the commercial behavioral program, which provides several options for obtaining support for behavior change.[65]

The commercial program has several different program offerings as summarized in Figure 3.3. These include 11-week "Engage" groups or individual programs that have a 1-hour weekly group meeting with a nutrition and weight management

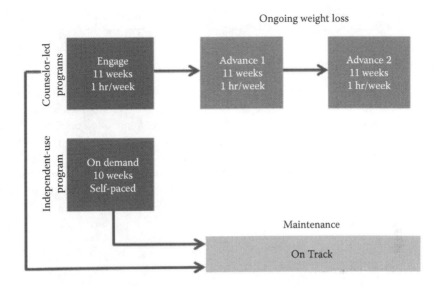

FIGURE 3.3   iDiet program offerings. (Adapted from iDiet. Available from: www.theidiet.com)

education unit supporting iDiet principles together with opportunities for support and discussion. Participants can also communicate with their counselor and other participants in their group via a website message board, and are encouraged (but not required) to log their weight in an individual dashboard, which illustrates progress graphically for the participant and can be seen by their counselor. Each group program runs as a closed group, that is, with members remaining within their assigned group for the full 11 weeks, and is led by a counselor who completed a group leadership training program and typically has a background in dietetics or health coaching. Individuals wishing to continue beyond their initial program can sign up for a second 11-week "Advance" program or can transition to low-intensity On Track website options that rely on moderated message boards for communication.

A unique feature of the counselor-led iDiet programs is that they are implemented through an online videoconference meeting (groups of up to 15 participants), as well as in-person meetings (groups of up to 20 participants). A recent analysis of results in the commercial program[1] reported no significant difference in percent weight loss between videoconference and in-person programs, and videoconference programs also have an increased percentage of participants reporting their weight on the website. As noted in the analysis,[1] in-person programs have long been considered the gold-standard for behavioral treatment of people with obesity,[66] but this modality has inherent burdens such as travel time and cost for both enrollees and counselors. The Das et al.[1] analysis is the first comparison of videoconference and in-person weight loss programs in adults, and notes that the videoconferencing option can be performed with smartphones, tablets, or computers, and can therefore be used for routine implementation of lower-burden weight loss programs in diverse locations.

In addition to the counselor-led programs, an asynchronous On Demand program is offered to allow independent program use, in which participants receive education modules via their website dashboard for self-paced use and communicate via moderated message boards with trained counselors and other independent program users.

TYPICAL MENU PLAN

Participants in the behavioral iDiet program are provided with an EasyPlan menu of self-selection food choices that either have recipes or are construction meals that can be created out of foods purchased in supermarkets that do not need cooking. There are food choices for people who eat meat as well as vegetarians and vegans. Similar menus are provided in the iDiet book. Each participant is assigned a menu calorie level designed to create a 500–1000 kcal/day reduction in energy intake compared to usual energy requirements, and portion sizes for meals and snacks are given along with recipes. The following menu is an example for a typical day for an individual assigned to a 1200 kcal/day menu.

BREAKFAST: Choose one per meal

1 egg fried/boiled/poached + 1 ½ slices high-fiber toast with 1 tsp butter + 1 cup fresh fruit

1/2 cup or more high-fiber cereal with 1 T each of nuts & raisins + 1/2 cup 0% plain Greek
  yogurt + 1/2 cup fresh fruit

MID-MORNING SNACK: Choose one per snack

1/2 cup high-fiber cereal + 1/2 cup milk + 1/4 cup berries

2 sticks light string cheese

LUNCH: Choose one per meal

1 cup thick, non-creamy soup such as lentil or beef barley + 1 small orange + 2 T peanuts

Soup & Sandwich: 1 cup broth vegetable soup + 1 ham sandwich made with 2 slices iDiet legal bread,
  2 thin slices ham, 1 slice fat free cheese, 1 tsp low-cal mayo, mustard, lettuce, tomato, onion,
  hot peppers

MID-AFTERNOON SNACK: Choose one per snack

4 sticks celery + 1 T peanut butter, or 4 sticks celery + 1/2 cup low-fat cottage cheese

1 medium apple + 4 pecan halves

DINNER: Choose one per meal

4 oz. grilled skinless chicken breast warmed w/ 1/4 cups tomato sauce and 1 T grated parmesan + 1 ½
  cups cooked green veggies w/ 1/4 tsp butter + side salad with drizzle of olive oil & vinegar or 1 tsp
  low-cal dressing

1 veggie burger patty + 1 high-fiber roll, with condiments of choice (mustard and/or ketchup) + 2 cups
  mixed garden salad with drizzle of olive oil & vinegar or 2 tsp low-calorie dressing

DESSERT: Choose one per meal

Ice Cream Sundae: 1/4 cup sugar free ice cream + 1/2 cup high-fiber cereal

Chocolate-Tipped Strawberries and Cream: 1 cup strawberries + 1 ½ square (~15 g) bittersweet
  chocolate + 1/4 cup light whipped cream (optional)

WHAT MAKES THE iDIET EFFECTIVE?

In contrast to most previous studies,[67–71] participants in the iDiet program report a significant decrease in hunger as illustrated in Figure 3.4. In addition, high hunger at baseline and a decrease in hunger during program participation are significant predictors of the magnitude of weight loss even when other eating behavior variables are

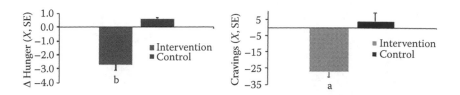

FIGURE 3.4 Changes in hunger and food cravings in iDiet intervention participants in a randomized trial, compared to weight listed controls over six months. Between group difference measured by GLM (general linear model) adjusting for baseline score of the variable, age, and sex. Significant P values are indicated by the letters a (P < 0.05) and b (P < 0.01). (Data from Batra P. et al. *Obesity* 2013;21(11):2256–63; Batra P. et al. *Appetite* 2013;69:1–7.)

included in the same model.[11] Although hunger is a basic drive indicating the need for food, in the context of weight loss, hunger suppression is beneficial and these data suggest that the iDiet prioritization of hunger suppression via dietary composition and use of free foods is an effective program strategy contributing to program success.[11]

In addition, and unlike most behavioral programs, use of the iDiet program is associated with a reduction in both the frequency and severity of food cravings[12] (Figure 3.3). Most individuals with overweight or obesity experience food cravings, that are typically for high-caloric foods in general, and sweets, carbohydrates, and fast food specifically,[72-74] and food cravings have been suggested to be both an impediment to weight loss and a promoter of recidivism after weight loss.[75-77] Thus, the effect of iDiet on reducing food cravings likely contributes to program success. However, it is noteworthy that while both hunger and food cravings are included in models predicting weight loss on iDiet, only hunger is a significant predictor. This suggests that cravings may be a conditioned sensation promoted by hunger that is acquired by repeated experience of eating the craved food in a non-satiated state,[74,78,79] and further suggests that the reduction in hunger with iDiet is a more fundamental determinant of program effectiveness, with the reduction in cravings being a secondary consequence of changes in hunger.

A pilot study also provided the first demonstration and localization of beneficial changes in the brain's reward system activity that was potentially influenced by a behavioral weight loss program. The pilot was a 6-month randomized controlled trial of the intervention versus a wait-listed control. The identified areas were involved in anticipation and reception of reward.[80] Furthermore, as described by Deckersbach et al.[80] and summarized in Figure 3.5, the study also provided the first demonstration of significant changes in *relative* reward system activation—that is, decreased activation for high-calorie foods and increased activation for low-calorie foods. While the regulation of food intake via the reward system is clearly complicated,[81] the fact that changes were identified in both the dorsal and the ventral striatum suggested broad changes occurred in reward system responsiveness, which potentially impacts the valuation of different foods both at the level of anticipation of consumption and at the level of actual consumption.[80,82] These findings indicate that participants in the iDiet program experience

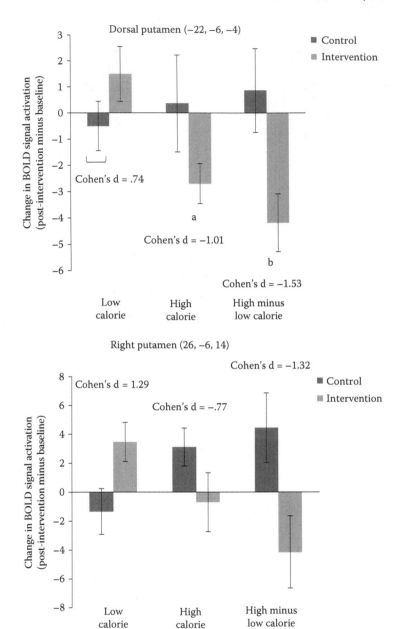

FIGURE 3.5 Differences between groups in changes over time (baseline to six months) in blood oxygen-level-dependent (BOLD) signal 16). p-values (max-voxels) for high-calorie (HC) and low-calorie (LC) foods minus non-food (NF) paired images, and changes in relative signal strength for HC and LC (delta values for HC-NF minus LC-NF): significance is denoted with the letter a (P < 0.05) or b (P < 0.01), and relevant Cohen's d-values are given as numerals.

a relative devaluation of anticipated reward for eating high-calorie foods that are easy to overeat combined with amplified anticipated reward for eating the low-calorie foods that support weight loss. Such alterations could potentially underlie both general program effectiveness and the reported changes in hunger and food cravings. However, it should be noted these results were obtained on a relatively small number of subjects (n = 13) and further work is needed to evaluate these initial findings.

CARDIOMETABOLIC CHANGES ON THE iDIET PROGRAM

As expected, the 8% mean weight loss in the iDiet clinical trial was accompanied by significant improvements in most measured cardiometabolic risk factors, including fasting serum total cholesterol (TC), LDL-C, non-high-density lipoprotein cholesterol (non-HDL-C), TC/HDL ratio, glucose concentrations, and systolic and diastolic blood pressures[15] (Table 3.2). There was also a significant improvement in reported health-related quality of life. Given that mean weight loss was of a greater magnitude than that achieved in the Diabetes Prevention Program,[17] and with a recent report showing greater weight loss from the commercial iDiet program (13.5%), it is likely that iDiet has the potential for even greater effects on cardiometabolic risk factors, including attenuating and reversing new diagnoses of diabetes; however, there are currently no published research studies evaluating these additional benefits.[1]

ONGOING RESEARCH

The iDiet is a relatively new weight loss program and ongoing studies in community groups, worksites, and military families will provide further data on the effectiveness of the program in different population groups.

PROS AND CONS OF USING THE iDIET PROGRAM

No weight loss program is "easy" in the sense that changing the dietary habits built up over a lifetime is more difficult than continuing current eating habits. Motivation for weight loss is, therefore, a necessary prerequisite for success in all weight loss programs, including iDiet. Nevertheless, the low dropout rate and high mean weight loss of the behavioral iDiet program compared to conventional behavioral programs suggests that iDiet is highly acceptable to enrollees.

THE PROS: EXCEPTIONAL RESULTS, FLEXIBLE FOOD PLANS, REDUCED HUNGER AND CRAVINGS, AND NO REQUIREMENT FOR FOOD LOGGING

Mean weight loss in the behavioral iDiet program is high compared to conventional behavioral programs and dropout rate is low, suggesting that the majority of enrollees will lose clinically impactful amounts of weight. The program appears to work over a broad demographic, being effective across a range of socioeconomic circumstances and among different racial and ethnic groups. Food plans are flexible and

TABLE 3.2

Body Weight and Cardiometabolic Risk Factors of Participants Completing the Weight Loss Program and Wait-Listed Control

Outcome Measure	Weight Loss Program	Wait-Listed	P Value[a]
Weight, kg	n = 83[b]	n = 34	
Baseline	93.6 ± 2.3	90.2 ± 3.9	
6 month	85.7 ± 2.0	91.1 ± 4.2	
Difference (6 month—baseline)	−8.0 ± 0.7	0.9 ± 0.5	<0.0001
BMI, kg/m²	n = 83[b]	n = 34	
Baseline	33.3 ± 0.7	33.3 ± 1.2	
6 month	30.5 ± 0.6	33.6 ± 1.3	
Difference (6 month—baseline)	−2.8 ± 0.2	0.3 ± 0.2	<0.0001
Systolic BP, mm Hg	n = 74	n = 27	
Baseline	132.25 ± 2.11	124.69 ± 2.01	
6 month	123.74 ± 1.89	130.19 ± 2.69	
Difference (6 month—baseline)	−8.51 ± 1.47	5.50 ± 2.08	<0.0001
Diastolic BP, mm Hg	n = 74	n = 27	
Baseline	83.56 ± 1.28	81.70 ± 1.94	
6 month	75.42 ± 1.23	81.20 ± 2.05	
Difference (6 month—baseline)	−8.14 ± 1.27	−0.50 ± 1.28	<0.001
Total Cholesterol, mg/dl	n = 72	n = 25	
Baseline	196.68 ± 3.81	196.12 ± 9.11	
6 month	183.47 ± 4.25	196.88 ± 8.67	
Difference (6 month—baseline)	−13.21 ± 2.95	0.76 ± 3.74	0.01
LDL-C, mg/dl	n = 68	n = 20	
Baseline	125.35 ± 3.65	133.05 ± 6.75	
6 month	111.88 ± 3.79	128.35 ± 6.60	
Difference (6 month—baseline)	−13.47 ± 2.67	−4.70 ± 3.94	0.05
HDL-C, mg/dl	n = 72	n = 25	
Baseline	47.18 ± 1.82	53.48 ± 3.49	
6 month	49.29 ± 1.78	54.76 ± 3.94	
Difference (6 month—baseline)	2.11 ± 0.87	1.28 ± 1.34	0.96
Non HDL-C, mg/dl	n = 66	n = 23	
Baseline	148.61 ± 3.80	149.39 ± 8.28	
6 month	134.20 ± 4.10	148.13 ± 7.85	
Difference (6 month—baseline)	−14.41 ± 2.86	−1.26 ± 3.79	0.01
Triglycerides, mg/dl	n = 72	n = 25	
Baseline	128.57 ± 7.04	106.96 ± 10.93	
6 month	121.13 ± 7.56	109.56 ± 13.77	
Difference (6 month—baseline)	−7.44 ± 6.94	2.60 ± 7.25	0.77
Total cholesterol/HDL-C Ratio	n = 72	n = 23	
Baseline	4.54 ± 0.17	4.06 ± 0.23	

(Continued)

TABLE 3.2 (*Continued*)

Body Weight and Cardiometabolic Risk Factors of Participants Completing the Weight Loss Program and Wait-Listed Control

Outcome Measure	Weight Loss Program	Wait-Listed	P Value[a]
6 month	3.98 ± 0.14	3.97 ± 0.23	
Difference (6 month—baseline)	−0.56 ± 0.09	−0.10 ± 0.12	0.05
Glucose, mg/dl	n = 73	n = 26	
Baseline	100.97 ± 1.59	106.85 ± 7.86	
6 month	94.60 ± 1.28	113.15 ± 10.52	
Difference (6 month—baseline)	−6.37 ± 1.55	6.31 ± 3.55	<0.001

Source: Adapted from reference Salinardi TC. et al. *American Journal of Clinical Nutrition* 2013;97(4):667–676.

[a] P values for baseline and 6 month weights were calculated using log transformed values. Weight difference calculated using the log of the ratio (6 month/baseline weight). Transformation of other variables was not required.

[b] One intervention participant completed the weight loss program but was not available for weight measurements.

Values are reported as means ± SEM.

SI conversion factors: To convert total cholesterol, LDL-C, HDL-C, and non HDL-C values from mg/dL to mmol/L, multiply by 0.0259; triglyceride values from mg/dL to mmol/L, by 0.0113; glucose values from mg/dL to mmol/L by 0.0555.

include options for people who eat meat, vegetarians, vegans, and those who are lactose intolerant. The results are achieved without an essential requirement for logging food or increasing exercise, which are likely to be important benefits for some individuals with overweight and obesity. The documented hunger suppression and reduced food cravings are program benefits that are likely to be appreciated by participants and contribute to program success.

The Cons: Initial Requirement for High Adherence to Provided Menus

As iDiet strongly recommends the use of self-selection menu items and recipes, it is more "prescriptive" than programs such as the Diabetes Prevention Program, which allow individuals to consume any foods of their choice and implement calorie restriction via food logging and prioritization of low fat/low energy density food choices. This feature may be a disadvantage for some individuals needing to lose weight who prefer to use their own foods. Although the menu items are broad and include typical foods that are popular, participants are discouraged from using their own recipes and food brands in the initial weeks while weight loss patterns are established.

In addition, the one subgroup for which the iDiet program has been found to be relatively less successful is adults under 30 years, as observed through lower enrollment rates, lower percentage continuing to report their weight to 11 weeks, and lower weight loss (mean percent weight loss, 5.5%) compared to older age groups.[1] Although mean weight loss is still in the clinically impactful range and greater than that of other behavioral programs reporting data by age group,[83,84] young adults may see less success from program results compared to older adults. The reasons behind these findings remain unknown, but younger adults may have a more difficult time with menu adherence and resisting outside social pressures, making it harder to adhere to behavioral weight loss programs in general.

IS THE iDIET RIGHT FOR YOUR PATIENT?

The iDiet is a healthy eating plan designed for sustainable weight loss, and is generally consistent with Institute of Medicine guidelines for nutritional adequacy and health. It is currently only recommended for use in adults, and there are no data for individuals under 20 years of age. There are a few factors that should be considered for patients considering the program.

1. The overarching goal of iDiet is to make sustainable changes to the patient's eating patterns that will result in sustainable weight loss. This is achieved through initial high adherence to self-selection menu plans, which are generally broadly flexible but do not include every specific food a particular patient may want. The program, therefore, necessarily restricts food choices and requires the willingness of individuals to be flexible about what they eat during the intensive initial phase of the program.
2. The program does not require food logging, which is likely to be a very positive feature for individuals who have previously tried to log their food and found that it is too burdensome to sustain.
3. The program also does not essentially require exercise, which again may be a positive feature for individuals who are sedentary or have limitations to what exercise they can do.
4. The program has options for vegetarians and vegans as well as those who are lactose intolerant. However, because high fiber is a central component of the program, individuals who are following a gluten-free diet may find the menu choices restrictive.

REFERENCES

1. Das SK, Brown C, Urban LE, O'Toole J, Gamache MMG, Weerasekara YK, Roberts SB. Weight loss in videoconference and in-person iDiet weight loss programs in worksites and community groups. *Obesity* 2017; 25(6):1033–41.
2. Jensen MD, Ryan DH, Apovian CM. et al. 2013 AHA/ACC/TOS guideline for the management of overweight and obesity in adults: A report of the American College of Cardiology/American Heart Association Task Force on Practice Guidelines and The Obesity Society. *J Am Coll Cardiol* 2014;63(25 Pt B):2985–3023.
3. Cefalu WT, Bray GA, Home PD. et al. Advances in the science, treatment, and prevention of the disease of obesity: Reflections from a diabetes care editors' expert forum. *Diabetes Care* 2015;38(8):1567–82.

4. Dunkley AJ, Bodicoat DH, Greaves CJ, Russell C, Yates T, Davies MJ, Khunti K. Diabetes prevention in the real world: Effectiveness of pragmatic lifestyle interventions for the prevention of type 2 diabetes and of the impact of adherence to guideline recommendations: A systematic review and meta-analysis. *Diabetes Care* 2014;37(4):922–33.

5. Jolly K, Lewis A, Beach J, Denley J, Adab P, Deeks JJ, Daley A, Aveyard P. Comparison of range of commercial or primary care led weight reduction programmes with minimal intervention control for weight loss in obesity: Lighten Up randomised controlled trial. *BMJ (Clinical Research Edition)* 2011;343:d6500.

6. Madigan CD, Daley AJ, Lewis AL, Jolly K, Aveyard P. Which weight-loss programmes are as effective as Weight Watchers(R)?: Non-inferiority analysis. *Br J Gen Pract* 2014;64(620):e128–36.

7. Little P, Stuart B, Hobbs FR. et al. An internet-based intervention with brief nurse support to manage obesity in primary care (POWeR+): A pragmatic, parallel-group, randomised controlled trial. *Lancet Diabetes Endocrinol* 2016;4(10):821–8.

8. Gudzune KA, Doshi RS, Mehta AK, Chaudhry ZW, Jacobs DK, Vakil RM, Lee CJ, Bleich SN, Clark JM. Efficacy of commercial weight-loss programs: An updated systematic review. *Ann Intern Med* 2015;162(7):501–12. Epub 2015/04/07.

9. Booth HP, Prevost TA, Wright AJ, Gulliford MC. Effectiveness of behavioural weight loss interventions delivered in a primary care setting: A systematic review and meta-analysis. *Fam Pract* 2014;31(6):643–53.

10. Johnston BC, Kanters S, Bandayrel K. et al. Comparison of weight loss among named diet programs in overweight and obese adults: A meta-analysis. *JAMA* 2014;312(9):923–33.

11. Batra P, Das SK, Salinardi T, Robinson L, Saltzman E, Scott T, Pittas AG, Roberts SB. Eating behaviors as predictors of weight loss in a 6 month weight loss intervention. *Obesity* 2013;21(11):2256–63.

12. Batra P, Das SK, Salinardi T, Robinson L, Saltzman E, Scott T, Pittas AG, Roberts SB. Relationship of cravings with weight loss and hunger. Results from a 6 month worksite weight loss intervention. *Appetite* 2013;69:1–7.

13. Keys A, Brozek J, Henschel A, Mickelson O, Taylor H. *The Biology of Human Starvation*. Minneapolis: University of Minnesota Press; 1950.

14. Wansink B, Tal A, Shimizu M. First foods most: After 18-hour fast, people drawn to starches first and vegetables last. *Arch Intern Med* 2012;172(12):961–3.

15. Salinardi TC, Batra P, Roberts SB, Urban LE, Robinson LM, Pittas AG, Lichtenstein AH, Deckersbach T, Saltzman E, Das SK. Lifestyle intervention reduces body weight and improves cardiometabolic risk factors in worksites. *Am J Clin Nutr* 2013;97(4):667–76.

16. Deckersbach T, Das SK, Urban LE, Salinardi T, Batra P, Rodman AM, Arulpragasam AR, Dougherty DD, Roberts SB. Pilot randomized trial demonstrating reversal of obesity-related abnormalities in reward system responsivity to food cues with a behavioral intervention. *Nutr Diabetes* 2014;4:e129.

17. Knowler WC, Barrett-Connor E, Fowler SE, Hamman RF, Lachin JM, Walker EA, Nathan DM. Reduction in the incidence of type 2 diabetes with lifestyle intervention or metformin. *N Engl J Med* 2002;346(6):393–403.

18. Ahern AL, Olson AD, Aston LM, Jebb SA. Weight Watchers on prescription: An observational study of weight change among adults referred to Weight Watchers by the NHS. *BMC Public Health* 2011;11:434.

19. Dansinger ML, Gleason JA, Griffith JL, Selker HP, Schaefer EJ. Comparison of the Atkins, Ornish, Weight Watchers, and Zone diets for weight loss and heart disease risk reduction: A randomized trial. *JAMA* 2005;293(1):43–53. PubMed PMID: 15632335.

20. Wing RR, Crane MM, Thomas JG, Kumar R, Weinberg B. Improving weight loss outcomes of community interventions by incorporating behavioral strategies. *Am J Public Health* 2010;100(12):2513–9.

21. Wing RR, Tate DF, Gorin AA, Raynor HA, Fava JL. A self-regulation program for maintenance of weight loss. *N Engl J Med* 2006;355(15):1563–71.
22. Wing RR. Treatment options for obesity: Do commercial weight loss programs have a role? *JAMA* 2010;304(16):1837–8.
23. Klem ML, Wing RR, McGuire MT, Seagle HM, Hill JO. A descriptive study of individuals successful at long-term maintenance of substantial weight loss. *Am J Clin Nutr* 1997;66(2):239–46.
24. McGuire MT, Wing RR, Klem ML, Lang W, Hill JO. What predicts weight regain in a group of successful weight losers? *J Consult Clin Psychol* 1999;67(2):177–85.
25. Kruger J, Blanck HM, Gillespie C. Dietary and physical activity behaviors among adults successful at weight loss maintenance. *Int J Behav Nutr Phys Act* 2006;3:17.
26. Wadden TA, Volger S, Sarwer DB. et al. A two-year randomized trial of obesity treatment in primary care practice. *N Engl J Med* 2011;365(21):1969–79.
27. Phelan S, Liu T, Gorin A, Lowe M, Hogan J, Fava J, Wing RR. What distinguishes weight-loss maintainers from the treatment-seeking obese? Analysis of environmental, behavioral, and psychosocial variables in diverse populations. *Ann Behav Med* 2009;38(2):94–104.
28. Hindle L, Carpenter C. An exploration of the experiences and perceptions of people who have maintained weight loss. *J Hum Nutr Diet: Journal of the British Dietetic Association* 2011;24(4):342–50.
29. Del Corral P, Bryan DR, Garvey WT, Gower BA, Hunter GR. Dietary adherence during weight loss predicts weight regain. *Obesity* 2011;19(6):1177–81.
30. Linde JA, Jeffery RW, French SA, Pronk NP, Boyle RG. Self-weighing in weight gain prevention and weight loss trials. *Ann Behav Med* 2005;30(3):210–6.
31. Williamson DA, Anton SD, Han H. et al. Early behavioral adherence predicts short and long-term weight loss in the POUNDS LOST study. *J Behav Med* 2010;33(4):305–14.
32. Funk KL, Stevens VJ, Appel LJ. et al. Associations of internet website use with weight change in a long-term weight loss maintenance program. *J Med Internet Res* 2010;12(3):e29.
33. Wang X, Lyles MF, You T, Berry MJ, Rejeski WJ, Nicklas BJ. Weight regain is related to decreases in physical activity during weight loss. *Med Sci Sports Exerc* 2008;40(10):1781–8.
34. Reyes NR, Oliver TL, Klotz AA, Lagrotte CA, Vander Veur SS, Virus A, Bailer BA, Foster GD. Similarities and differences between weight loss maintainers and regainers: A qualitative analysis. *J Acad Nutr Diet* 2012;112(4):499–505.
35. Locke EA, Latham GP. *A Theory of Goal Setting & Task Performance*. Englewood Cliffs, NJ. Prentice Hall; 1990.
36. Smith CF, Williamson DA, Womble LG, Johnson J, Burke LE. Psychometric development of a multidimensional measure of weight-related attitudes and behaviors. *Eating and Weight Disorders* 2000;5(2):73–86.
37. Bandura A. *Social Foundation of Thought and Action: A Social Cognitive Theory*. Englewood Cliffs, NJ: Prentice Hall; 1986.
38. Foreyt JP, Poston WS, 2nd. The role of the behavioral counselor in obesity treatment. *J Am Diet Assoc* 1998;98(10 Suppl 2):S27–30.
39. Jenkins DJ, Wolever TM, Taylor RH. et al. Glycemic index of foods: A physiological basis for carbohydrate exchange. *Am J Clin Nutr* 1981;34:362–6.
40. Karl JP, Roberts SB. Energy density, energy intake, and body weight regulation in adults. *Advances in Nutrition*. 2014;5(6):835–50.
41. Institute of Medicine. *Dietary Reference Intakes: The Essential Guide to Nutrient Requirements*. Washington, D.C.: National Academy of Sciences; 2006.
42. Jenkins DA, Jones PH, Lamarche B. et al. Effect of a dietary portfolio of cholesterol-lowering foods given at 2 levels of intensity of dietary advice on serum lipids in hyperlipidemia: A randomized controlled trial. *JAMA* 2011;306(8):831–9.

43. Roberts SB. High glycemic index foods, hunger and obesity: Is there a connection? *Nutr Reviews* 2000;58:163–9.
44. Eisenstein JK, Roberts SB, Dallal GE, Saltzman E. High-protein weight-loss diets: Are they safe and do they work? A review of the experimental and epdemiological data. *Nutr Rev* 2002;60:189–200.
45. Yao M, Roberts SB. Dietary energy density and weight regulation. *Nutr Rev* 2001;59:247–57.
46. Howarth NC, Saltzman E, Roberts SB. Dietary fiber and weight regulation. *Nutr Rev* 2001;59:129–39.
47. Gilhooly CH, Das SK, Golden JK. et al. Use of cereal fiber to facilitate adherence to a human caloric restriction program. *Aging Clin Exp Res* 2008;20(6):513–20.
48. Slavin JL. Dietary fiber and body weight. *Nutrition* 2005;21(3):411–8.
49. Halton TL, Hu FB. The effects of high protein diets on thermogenesis, satiety and weight loss: A critical review. *J Am Coll Nutr* 2004;23(5):373–85.
50. McCrory MA, Burke A, Roberts SB. Dietary (sensory) variety and energy balance. *Physiol Behav.* 2012;107(4):576–83.
51. Foster GD, Wyatt HR, Hill JO, McGuckin BG, Brill C, Mohammed BS. A randomized trial of a low-carbohydrate diet for obesity. *N Engl J Med* 2003;348(21):2082–90.
52. Sacks FM, Bray GA, Carey VJ. et al. Comparison of weight-loss diets with different compositions of fat, protein and carbohydrates. *N Engl J Med* 2009;360:859–73.
53. Das SK, Gilhooly CH, Golden JK. et al. Long-term effects of 2 energy-restricted diets differing in glycemic load on dietary adherence, body composition, and metabolism in CALERIE, a 1-year randomized controlled trial. *Am J Clin Nutr* 2007;85:1023–30.
54. Thomas DE, Elliott EJ, Baur L. Low glycaemic index or low glycaemic load diets for overweight and obesity. *Cochrane Database Syst Rev* 2007,(3):Cd005105. Epub 2007/07/20.
55. The Diabetes Prevention Program Research G. The Diabetes Prevention Program (DPP): Description of lifestyle intervention. *Diabetes Care* 2002;25(12):2165–71.
56. Berthoud HR, Morrison C. The brain, appetite, and obesity. *Annu Rev Psychol* 2008;59:55–92.
57. Roberts SB, Urban LE, Das SK. Effects of dietary composition on energy regulation: Consideration of multiple versus single dietary factor models. *Physiol Behav* 2014;(134):5.
58. Pittas A, Das SK, Hadjuk CL, Fuss P, Saltzman E, Roberts SB. A low-glycemic load diet facilitates greater weight loss in overweight adults with high insulin secretion but not in overweight adults with low insulin secretion in the CALERIE trial. *Diabetes Care* 2005;28:2939–41.
59. Ebbeling CB, Swain JF, Feldman HA, Wong WW, Hachey DL, Garcia-Lago E, Ludwig DS. Effects of dietary composition on energy expenditure during weight-loss maintenance. *JAMA* 2012;307(24):2627–34.
60. McNabb WL, Quinn MT, Rosing LS. Weight loss program for inner-city black women with non-insulin-dependent diabetes mellitus: Pathways. *J Am Diet Assoc* 1993;93:75–7.
61. Shintani TT, Hugher CK, Beckham S. Obesity and cardiovascular risk intervention through the ad libitum feeding of traditional Hawaiian diet. *Am J Clin Nutr* 1991;53:1647S–51S.
62. Patterson RE, Kristal AR, Glanz K, McLerran DF, Hebert JR, Heimendinger J, Linnan L, Probart C, Chamberlain RM. Components of the working well trial intervention associated with adoption of healthful diets. *Am J Prev Med* 1997;13(4):271–6.
63. Elder SJ, Roberts SB. The effects of exercise on food intake and body fatness: A summary of published studies. *Nutr Rev* 2007;65(1):1–19.
64. Roberts SB, Sargent BK. *The "I" Diet*. New York, NY. Workman Publishing; 2010.
65. iDiet. Available from: www.theidiet.com.
66. Kushner RF, Ryan DH. Assessment and lifestyle management of patients with obesity: Clinical recommendations from systematic reviews. *JAMA* 2014;312(9):943–52.

67. Dalle Grave R, Calugi S, Corica F, Di Domizio S, Marchesini G. Psychological variables associated with weight loss in obese patients seeking treatment at medical centers. *J Am Diet Assoc* 2009;109(12):2010–6.

68. Foster GD, Wadden TA, Swain RM, Stunkard AJ, Platte P, Vogt RA. The Eating Inventory in obese women: Clinical correlates and relationship to weight loss. *Int J Obes Relat Metab Disord* 1998;22(8):778–85.

69. McGuire MT, Jeffery RW, French SA, Hannan PJ. The relationship between restraint and weight and weight-related behaviors among individuals in a community weight gain prevention trial. *Int J Obes Relat Metab Disord* 2001;25(4):574–80.

70. Keranen AM, Savolainen MJ, Reponen AH, Kujari ML, Lindeman SM, Bloigu RS, Laitinen JH. The effect of eating behavior on weight loss and maintenance during a lifestyle intervention. *Prev Med* 2009;49(1):32–8.

71. Teixeira PJ, Silva MN, Coutinho SR, Palmeira AL, Mata J, Vieira PN, Carraca EV, Santos TC, Sardinha LB. Mediators of weight loss and weight loss maintenance in middle-aged women. *Obesity* 2010;18(4):725–35.

72. Delahanty L. Winning at losing: A guide to healthy weight loss. Meal replacements. Used correctly, weight-loss shakes and bars can offer nutritious options. *Diabetes Forecast* 2002;55(4):75–76, 8. Epub 2004/02/18.

73. Christensen L. Craving for sweet carbohydrate and fat-rich foods—possible triggers and impact on nutritional intake. *Nutrition Bulletin* 2007;32:43–51.

74. Gilhooly CH, Das SK, Golden JK, McCrory MA, Dallal GE, Saltzman E, Kramer FM, Roberts SB. Food cravings and energy regulation: The characteristics of craved foods and their relationship with eating behaviors and weight change during 6 months of dietary energy restriction. *Int J Obes* 2007;31(12):1849–58.

75. Sitton SC. Role of craving for carbohydrates upon completion of a protein-sparing fast. *Psychol Rep* 1991;69(2):683–6.

76. Forman EM, Hoffman KL, McGrath KB, Herbert JD, Brandsma LL, Lowe MR. A comparison of acceptance- and control-based strategies for coping with food cravings: An analog study. *Behav Res Ther* 2007;45(10):2372–86. Epub 2007/06/05.

77. Moreno S, Rodriguez S, Fernandez MC, Tamez J, Cepeda-Benito A. Clinical validation of the trait and state versions of the Food Craving Questionnaire. *Assessment* 2008;15(3):375–87.

78. Gibson EL, Desmond E. Chocolate craving and hunger state: Implications for the acquisition and expression of appetite and food choice. *Appetite* 1999;32(2):219–40.

79. Steel D, Kemps E, Tiggemann M. Effects of hunger and visuo-spatial interference on imagery-induced food cravings. *Appetite* 2006;46(1):36–40.

80. Deckersbach T, Das SK, Urban LE, Salinardi T, Batra P, Rodman AM, Arulpragasam AR, Dougherty DD, Roberts SB. Pilot randomized trial demonstrating reversal of obesity-related abnormalities in reward system responsivity to food cues with a behavioral intervention. *Nutr Diabetes* 2014;4:e129.

81. Carnell S, Gibson C, Benson L, Ochner CN, Geliebter A. Neuroimaging and obesity: Current knowledge and future directions. *Obes Rev: An Official Journal of the International Association for the Study of Obesity* 2012;13(1):43–56.

82. Stice E, Spoor S, Bohon C, Veldhuizen MG, Small DM. Relation of reward from food intake and anticipated food intake to obesity: A functional magnetic resonance imaging study. *J Abnorm Psychol* 2008;117(4):924–35.

83. Poobalan AS, Aucott LS, Precious E, Crombie IK, Smith WC. Weight loss interventions in young people (18–25 year olds): A systematic review. *Obes Rev* 2010;11(8):580–92.

84. Gokee-LaRose J, Gorin AA, Raynor HA, Laska MN, Jeffery RW, Levy RL, Wing RR. Are standard behavioral weight loss programs effective for young adults? *Int J Obes.* 2009;33(12):1374–80.

4 The Mediterranean Diet

Sally M. Cohen

CONTENTS

OVERVIEW

The Mediterranean Diet as we know it today emerged out of research conducted beginning in the late 1950s. The pivotal Seven Countries Study, led by influential health and nutrition researcher Ancel Keys, examined the relationship between diet and heart disease.[1] Keys and his team observed food consumption patterns and the prevalence of coronary heart disease across 16 cohorts in seven different countries: Greece, Italy, Spain, South Africa, Japan, Finland, and the United States. Their observations on the typical foods consumed in four of the study's cohorts—Crete and Corfu in Greece, Dalmatia in Croatia, and Montegiorgio in Italy—and the related low frequency of coronary heart disease in these countries, led to the identification of the Mediterranean Diet pattern and lifestyle.

According to their research, Keys and his team found that the Mediterranean Diet pattern differed from other traditional diets they studied in many ways. First, the Mediterranean Diet relied on olive oil as the main source of dietary fat. Additionally, intake of red meat was lower than in other cohorts, but consumption of seafood was relatively high. The Italian and Greek cohorts also consumed less dairy, but ate more fruits, vegetables, and grain products. In terms of nutrition, this meant that the Italian and Greek study subjects ate lower amounts of saturated fats, higher amounts of unsaturated fats, and nearly no trans fats. These subjects also had a high intake of fiber and phytochemicals including antioxidants due to the elevated levels of fruit, vegetable, and grain consumption. This plant-based way of eating, high in unsaturated fats, came to be known as the Mediterranean Diet. Ancel Keys promoted the Mediterranean Diet in his 1975 book, *How to eat well and stay well the Mediterranean way.*[2]

53

In the 1990s, Walter Willet and his team at Harvard University picked up the charge from Keys and further explored the virtues of the Mediterranean Diet.[3,4] In the midst of the low-fat diet craze, Willet's team began to expose the merits of the relatively higher fat Mediterranean Diet for the heart healthy benefits that Keys first identified. Willett's team also identified other health benefits associated with the Mediterranean, plant-based way of eating: lower rates of certain types of cancers, lower rates of cataracts, reduced prevalence of neurological birth defects known as neural tube defects, and lower rates of all-cause mortality.[5-7] At the time, Willett's research stirred up a lot of controversy among other doctors and researchers who felt that a lower fat diet was the best way to fight heart disease and obesity. Despite the scientific debate, the Mediterranean Diet began to gain traction among some health practitioners and health-conscious consumers.

Simultaneously, the Lyon Diet Heart Study reinforced previous findings related to the Mediterranean Diet's protective cardiovascular effect.[8] Michel de Lorgeril and team investigated the impact of the Mediterranean Diet on risk for myocardial infarction along with cardiac death and other composite cardiovascular outcomes. Their randomized, single-blind, secondary prevention trial was conducted among elderly French patients status-post a first myocardial infarction. The resulting data showed that a Mediterranean Diet significantly reduced the risk for recurrence of myocardial infarction and all-cause cardiovascular mortality amongst those patients following the prescribed Mediterranean Diet when compared with a control group that continued to follow their usual, healthy diet as prescribed by their doctor. Additionally, with an average of four years of follow-up, the Lyon Diet Heart Study was able to assess long-term compliance with the Mediterranean Diet after a shorter period (one year) of intervention. The research team found that, even after several years post-intervention, a majority of patients randomized into the Mediterranean Diet group continued to follow the eating pattern. This important finding reinforced the potential long-term impact of Mediterranean Diet education on patients' daily habits among a vulnerable, receptive population. Further, this finding validated the importance of nutrition counseling—used alone or in conjunction with prescription medications where appropriate—to create a lasting impact on health. Most importantly, it demonstrated the sheer stickiness of the Mediterranean Diet eating pattern in this population—for whatever reason patients chose to adhere to this way of eating for the long term.

Today, many other teams of researchers have studied the Mediterranean Diet pattern for its purported health benefits as well as for weight loss. While the Mediterranean Diet as we know it today remains true to the core plant-based tenets Keys identified more than half a century ago, the definition has been slightly expanded. In 1995, Oldways Preservation Trust, along with Willet's team at the Harvard School of Public Health and the World Health Organization, first released the Mediterranean Diet Pyramid to demonstrate the Mediterranean way of healthy eating.[9,10] The pyramid, still in use today, rests on a foundation of plant-based foods (vegetables, fruits, grains, beans, and legumes); includes fish and other seafood; small portions of dairy, poultry, and eggs; and even smaller portions of meat and sweet foods. It also includes wine in moderation, and makes a point to encourage regular physical activity and socialization around meal times. Oldways continues to promote the Mediterranean

Diet and its associated health benefits through the pyramid, various cookbooks, and other education materials that help healthcare practitioners counsel their patients on the Mediterranean Diet pattern, and help consumers follow this delicious way of eating.

Based in Barcelona, the Fundación Dieta Mediterránea (Mediterranean Diet Foundation) works to advance the Mediterranean Diet by ensuring continued research on the benefits of the eating pattern, distributing information stemming from research about the diet, and advocating for the dietary and lifestyle habits of Mediterranean populations.[11] Like Oldways, the Fundación Dieta Mediterránea has developed a diet pyramid reflecting the core tenets of the Mediterranean Diet. Also plant-based, the Fundación Dieta Mediterránea's pyramid sits on a foundation of whole grain carbohydrate foods like bread and pasta, as well as fruits and vegetables. The Fundación Dieta Mediterránea specifically advocates for half of the fruits and vegetables to be consumed raw. Olive oil is the main source of fat and the Fundación Dieta Mediterránea recommends consuming this fat at every meal. Plant-based sources of protein such as nuts and seeds, as well as low-sodium flavorings like garlic, onion, and herbs, and low-fat dairy should be consumed daily. The Fundación Dieta Mediterránea suggests consuming lean animal proteins—such as white meat, seafood, and eggs—as well as legumes and potatoes weekly. Sweets should be consumed sparingly and alcohol may be consumed in moderation accordingly with social and cultural beliefs. Fundación Dieta Mediterránea's pyramid also advocates that consumers take into account local customs, traditional food products, seasonality, sustainability, and biodiversity. The Fundación Dieta Mediterránea specifically promotes what they call "culinary activities" with a focus on preparing one's own meals rather than relying on pre-prepared, packaged, or restaurant foods. Like Oldways, the Fundación Dieta Mediterránea promotes physical activity and social interaction, but also notes the importance of adequate rest.

Though Ancel Keys brought global attention to the health benefits of the Mediterranean Diet in the 1950s and 1960s, inhabitants of countries like Croatia, Spain, Greece, Italy, Morocco, and Portugal have been preparing and enjoying Mediterranean Diet foods for centuries. And as both Oldways and the Fundación Dieta Mediterránea point out, the Mediterranean Diet is about more than just food—it is a long-standing lifestyle for people in many countries surrounding the Mediterranean Sea. Thus the Mediterranean Diet, as a way of life around food and eating, was formally recognized by UNESCO (The United Nations Educational, Scientific and Cultural Organization) by being inscribed on the Representative List of the Intangible Cultural Heritage of Humanity.[12] This designation recognizes traditions, passed on through generations, which contribute to the diversity of communities around the globe. Officially recognized in 2013, UNESCO acknowledges that the Mediterranean Diet is more than simply the foods eaten in the regions around the Mediterranean Sea. UNESCO also identifies the culturally-specific knowledge of farming, cooking, and sharing of food as crucial to the Mediterranean Diet way of life. Further, UNESCO recognizes the role of women—as the keepers and teachers of the Mediterranean Diet tradition—and the importance of perishable goods (i.e., open air) markets as a communal space for disseminating the ways of the Mediterranean Diet.

Just as UNESCO was recognizing the Mediterranean Diet for its cultural and historical significance, a new wave of research on the health benefits of the diet emerged out of a key Mediterranean region.[13] A Spanish team began publishing on the effects of the Mediterranean Diet on risk for chronic diseases as part of the PREDIMED (Prevención con Dieta Mediterránea) trial in 2011.[14] The primary prevention study investigated the risk for heart attack, stroke, and all-cause cardiac mortality among community-dwelling, middle-age, or older Spanish adults at high risk for, but without prior history of, cardiovascular disease. The team found dramatic and significant reductions in participants who followed a Mediterranean Diet supplemented with either olive oil or nuts, compared with those who followed a traditional low-fat diet. Subsequent secondary analyses of the PREDIMED data also showed significant reduction in risk for development of type 2 diabetes among the same Spanish subjects at high risk for cardiovascular disease who followed the Mediterranean Diet supplemented with extra virgin olive oil, compared with those following the low-fat diet.[15] A follow-up study, PREDIMED-Plus, began in 2013 to investigate the impact of the Mediterranean Diet on risk for cardiovascular disease among free-living Spanish subjects with overweight or obesity and metabolic syndrome.[16] Results from PREDIMED-Plus are still forthcoming at the time of this publication.

HOW THE DIET WORKS

Unlike many traditional weight loss diets, the Mediterranean Diet is less stringent—that is, less "eat this, don't eat that"—and more of an overall pattern of eating and lifestyle. As the Oldways Preservation Trust and Fundación Dieta Mediterránea pyramids showcase, the Mediterranean Diet includes all foods, though perhaps in proportions that are not aligned with current ways of eating in many parts of the Western World.[10,11] Because it is not a rigid program, the Mediterranean Diet can be difficult to "prescribe" to patients who wish to improve their health or lose weight. Because of the rather flexible guidelines of the Mediterranean Diet, the involvement of a Registered Dietitian may be helpful to guide a patient's transition from a typical Western diet to a Mediterranean eating pattern.

As previously reviewed, the Mediterranean Diet is plant-based—patients should expect to eat vegetables, fruits, and grains at each meal. The Mediterranean Diet's primary sources of protein are beans and legumes, as well as fish and other seafood, consumed multiple times per day, and complimented with small portions of low-fat dairy and eggs. Poultry and meat are infrequent inclusions in the Mediterranean Diet, and sweets even less often. Alcohol may be consumed in moderation and in accordance with the patient's cultural and social norms. Though regular consumption of alcohol—especially wine, which, in moderation, carries its own set of health benefits associated with phytochemical content—is customary in the regions from which the Mediterranean Diet first emerged, it is not a necessary inclusion for all patients adopting the eating pattern. While the Mediterranean Diet typically includes the types of produce, grains, and seafood available in and around the Mediterranean Sea, it can be easily adapted to the types of foods available in the patient's surroundings. According to the Fundación Dieta Mediterránea, the focus should be on minimally processed foods, prepared simply and without preservatives.[11] Locality and seasonality may or may not be important—while they are at the crux of the Mediterranean way of eating, they may not be feasible for patients living in food deserts or colder climates where fresh produce is not locally available year round. However, winter storing fruits and vegetables, as well as hardy greens, may substitute for other produce in the colder months. Further, frozen fruits and vegetables—nutritionally similar or even equivalent to fresh versions—may be used if fresh produce is not seasonally available or not within the patient's financial budget.

The Fundación Dieta Mediterránea stresses the importance of avoiding packaged, processed foods.[11] This stance makes sense from a health and weight loss perspective, as these foods are commonly high in sodium, sugar, and unhealthy fats—all of which may contribute to increased risks for hypertension, cardiovascular disease, diabetes, and weight gain. These foods are usually calorie-, but not nutrient-dense—in direct opposition to the types of foods included in the Mediterranean Diet. Moreover, they are often produced far away, from products that may or may not be grown in season, let alone grown from the ground (i.e., instead of in the lab). Similarly, the Mediterranean Diet does not explicitly include any beverages except water and wine. This means that juices, regular sodas, sweetened coffee and tea drinks, and other sugar-sweetened beverages—all major contributors of excess calories in the typical American diet—are technically "off limits" when following the Mediterranean Diet. Further, artificial sweeteners are not part of the Mediterranean Diet, ruling out diet soda, and any other beverages or foods sweetened with aspartame, saccharin, sucralose, accsulfame-K, added (not naturally-occurring) sugar alcohols, or even stevia. Due to the guidance regarding avoidance of highly processed foods, fast foods also are not technically included in the Mediterranean Diet—nor are commercially produced baked goods, frozen meals, or even most canned products. Exclusion of these types of foods from the Mediterranean Diet—and the inverse emphasis on fresh, minimally processed foods—represents a shift away from the typical American or Western diet, and a major counterpoint to the usual high intake of salt and added sugar. It also represents a shift toward increased intake of dietary fiber, and a move from unhealthy saturated fats toward heart-healthy unsaturated fats.

It is crucial to reiterate that, because the Mediterranean Diet is not actually a diet, but rather a dietary pattern—or, more accurately, a lifestyle—it does not simply address food. The Mediterranean Diet also addresses the role of general well-being and overall health—both physical and mental—as a part of a healthy lifestyle. It is difficult to disentangle the social aspects of the Mediterranean Diet from the culinary components. Consumption of meals surrounded by friends and family is deeply rooted in the Mediterranean culture as first noted by Ancel Keys and his team.[1,2] The habit of regularly eating with loved ones means that the act of food consumption is coupled closely with conversation and interpersonal connection. This likely contributes to health in multiple ways, including simply eating more slowly and lengthening meal times. This diet promotes "mindful eating"—improving feelings of satiety and fullness as the brain and hormones have more time to react to expansion of the stomach in the presence of food. It may also improve satisfaction with food, thanks to increased time to savor various flavors, textures, and tastes. Additionally, the crucial social interaction inherent in the Mediterranean Diet lifestyle likely contributes to overall well-being—thanks to regular interpersonal interaction and the feelings of support provided by frequent engagement with a social network—a benefit of the Mediterranean Diet that is alluded to in research. It is important to note that, while several studies have indicated an improved quality of life associated with adoption of the Mediterranean Diet, it is not clear whether this is related to consuming meals with friends and family, or related specifically to the foods of the Mediterranean Diet. Achieving this social aspect of the Mediterranean Diet means stepping away from the "go, go, go" mentality of many of today's Western societies and, more specifically, eschewing on-the-go eating. It means setting aside time to prepare, cook, and enjoy a lengthier meal with friends and family, which may require planning ahead and more attention to schedule.

Just as social interaction is key to the Mediterranean Diet lifestyle, so is physical activity. The Mediterranean populations observed by Keys and subsequent researchers did not simply ingest a healthy diet, they also incorporated regular movement into their day-to-day lives. For these initial subjects, the Mediterranean Diet lifestyle perhaps did not include exercise as we know it today—instead, it may have simply involved walking for transportation, engaging in manual labor, or the occasional involvement in sports. Today's proponent of the Mediterranean Diet, though, may be more likely to commute via car or train and go to work to sit all day at a desk. Thus, it is important to find ways to incorporate physical activity into the daily routine, whether this means finding a new way to commute (e.g., walking or via bicycle), setting aside time during the work day to engage in light physical activity, or planning regular exercise sessions. It may not be possible to live the more active lifestyle of the Greek, Croatian, and Italian subjects Keys and team first observed, but it is crucial to find ways to ensure that regular and frequent physical activity becomes a habit. For this aspect of a Mediterranean Diet lifestyle, working with an Exercise Physiologist or Certified Personal Trainer may be helpful for patients who are not already engaged in a routine of physical activity.

CURRENT RESEARCH

Research conducted on the Mediterranean Diet between the late 1950s and the mid-1990s suggests a protective effect of this lifestyle on cardiovascular health and mortality, as well as a reduced risk for type 2 diabetes.[15] What had not been made clear, though, is the effectiveness of the use of the Mediterranean Diet as a weight loss diet. A handful of studies conducted in the past decade have begun to investigate whether following a Mediterranean Diet could lead to significant weight loss, in addition to the noted health benefits already described. Many recent studies exploring the use of the Mediterranean Diet for weight management face a common limitation— namely, that weight loss is investigated as a secondary outcome, rarely a primary focus of the research. It is also crucial to note that, while the Mediterranean Diet pattern has been defined by Oldways Preservation Trust and the Fundación Dieta Mediterránea, the various studies can develop their intervention diet in many different ways.[10,11] For example, while one study may focus on the supplementation of olive oil or nuts to achieve increased intake of monounsaturated and omega-3 fatty acids, another study may emphasize increasing plant-based foods in the dict and reducing meats. Further, these studies may or may not include the physical activity or social aspect of the Mediterranean Diet lifestyle in their interventions. Most importantly, these studies may or may not restrict calorie intake among participants. These important differences in study design and their related outcomes impact the ability of clinicians to make concrete dietary recommendations to patients whose sole goal is weight loss via adoption of the Mediterranean Diet. They also reinforce the fact that the Mediterranean Diet is a comprehensive lifestyle comprised of many facets, not a prescriptive diet per se.

In 2008, Buckland and colleagues published a systematic review of 21 studies conducted between 2000 and 2007 that examined the impact of the Mediterranean Diet on the risk for overweight and obesity.[17] The review included both observational—cohort and cross-sectional designs—and intervention studies. The studies involved participants from Mediterranean-adjacent European countries—including Italy, Cyprus, Greece, Spain, and France—as well as European countries removed from the Mediterranean Sea (Germany), North American countries (United States and Canada), and Asian participants (Hong Kong). The participants' health status ranged from normal weight, healthy subjects to overweight or obese patients, or patients with a history of coronary heart disease; their ages ranged from university-aged to elderly. Interestingly, each study included in the review defined the Mediterranean Diet in their own, unique way, though most emphasized the importance of increasing plant-based foods, using olive oil as the main source of dietary fat, and decreasing intake of red meat. Some of the intervention studies included in the review also incorporated physical activity components, while others provided instruction in Mediterranean Diet-style cooking, while still others explicitly included weight loss counseling. The control diets used in the intervention studies also varied: from the participants' usual healthy diets, to prescribed low-fat diets, to standard of care treatment common for the area where patients resided. Some intervention studies explicitly included calorie restriction for both the control and treatment groups, while others did not. The included studies varied in their approach regarding the lifestyle aspects (e.g., social components of dining, daily physical activity, seasonality of foods, and emphasis on home cooked foods versus processed or prepared foods) of the Mediterranean Diet in their intervention or analysis. The length of follow-up for the cohort and intervention studies ranged from just three months to nine years. Ability to adjust for confounders also varied. Hence, there was significant variation in the studies the team analyzed, in every aspect of research design. Not surprisingly, Buckland and colleagues found mixed results from the 21 studies they analyzed. Some studies found significant reductions in body mass index (BMI) among those participants following the Mediterranean Diet, other studies found decreased rates of obesity that were not significant, and other studies still found that results varied by sex or age group, with some showing significant reductions in weight or BMI with adoption of the Mediterranean Diet and others showing null results.

Just three years later, in 2011, Esposito and colleagues conducted a meta-analysis to investigate any possible causal relationship between the Mediterranean Diet and body weight.[18] Their analysis included only randomized controlled trials. They evaluated 16 trials comprised of a total of 19 study arms, all of which investigated the impact of the Mediterranean Diet on body weight—change in body weight or body mass index—as either a primary or secondary outcome. None of the studies included in the meta-analysis were double-blinded. In total, the meta-analysis included 3,436 participants across the various studies—of these, just over half were randomized to the Mediterranean Diet (intervention or treatment) groups, and the remaining participants were randomized to control diets. Participants in the included studies were from the United States as well as European and Middle Eastern countries, both bordering the Mediterranean Sea (Italy, Spain, France, Israel, Greece) and further afield (Germany, the Netherlands). Participants ranged from healthy subjects, to those with a history of cardiovascular disease, to others with obesity or obesity paired with other comorbidities (e.g., type 2 diabetes). The studies were conducted between 1994 and 2010. The study designs included both parallel and cross-over trials, with follow-up length ranging from eight weeks to five years. As with Buckland and colleague's systematic review, definitions of the Mediterranean Diet varied across the 16 studies from a focus on plant-based foods, to a focus on types of dietary fats, to inclusion of alcohol consumption. Similarly, some of the studies included physical activity components or calorie restriction, while others did not. Further, definitions of the control group diets ranged from low fat, to defined Acceptable Macronutrient Distribution Ranges, to energy restricted diets, to general healthy diets as advised by physicians and dietitians. Given the inconsistency in defining the Mediterranean Diet interventions, the control diets, and other aspects of the treatment protocol, it is not surprising that results from the 16 studies varied widely, from favoring the Mediterranean Diet for weight loss to favoring the control diet instead. Even within the same study, for example, different arms that compared the Mediterranean Diet to slightly different control diets (e.g., low fat or low carbohydrate), found conflicting results on whether the Mediterranean Diet was or was not superior to the control diet in terms of weight management. The analysis conducted by Esposito and colleagues concluded in favor of the Mediterranean Diet's impact on both weight (changes in body weight in kilograms) and body mass index, both with statistically significant results. The authors suggest that the Mediterranean Diet, coupled with calorie restriction, lead to a greater reduction in body weight and BMI.

More recently, a group of researchers in Spain led by Gomez-Huelgas set out to determine the impact of a Mediterranean lifestyle intervention on metabolic syndrome among Spanish participants.[19] The results of their randomized controlled trial were published in 2015, and body weight and BMI were included as secondary outcomes. Participants ranged in age from 18 to 80 years of age and were screened for metabolic syndrome—overweight or obesity were not criteria for inclusion in the study as long as the participants had markers of metabolic syndrome. The intervention lasted three years and the participants were randomized to either a Mediterranean Diet lifestyle intervention group or a control group. The Mediterranean Diet lifestyle intervention group was instructed on a plant-based diet with the use of olive oil for dietary fat—recommended number of servings per day or week of each food group were provided. Participants in the intervention group with overweight or obesity (as defined by body mass index) were instructed to restrict calorie intake. The intervention also included specific physical activity recommendations, and this group received intensive clinical visits with instruction on the components of the Mediterranean Diet, including provision of healthy recipes, instruction on types of physical activity, and types of dietary fat. The control group received standard of care treatment, with clinical visits focused on heart-healthy eating, increased physical activity, and recommended weight loss. The researchers found an improvement in several markers for metabolic syndrome—including statistically significant differences in change in waist circumference and both systolic and diastolic blood pressures—in the Mediterranean Diet lifestyle intervention group when compared with the control group. However, they did not find any statistically significant differences in the changes in body weight or body mass index between the two groups, and, in fact, less than 20% of participants in either group lost greater than 5% of initial body weight by the end of the study. On average, participants in both the Mediterranean Diet lifestyle intervention group and the control group gained weight (up to +0.9 kilograms) and saw an increase in body mass index (up to +0.31 kg/m^2) over the course of the study. The findings from this study have several key limitations that should be noted, including a high rate of participant dropout (>30% of participants did not complete the study) and lack of participant compliance with both calorie restriction and exercise recommendations. Further, the researchers did not stratify their results by body mass index, so it is not possible to say whether their Mediterranean Diet lifestyle intervention may have been more effective in terms of weight loss for specifically overweight or obese participants. Of note, though, most participants in the Mediterranean Diet lifestyle intervention group demonstrated a high level of adherence to the prescribed Mediterranean Diet, both during the intervention itself and even after three years of follow-up. After three years, these participants also had significantly improved quality of life scores, increased levels of physical activity, decreased daily calorie intake, and increased intake of heart healthy fats when compared with control group participants.

In 2016, Mancini and colleagues published a systematic review of five randomized controlled trials that explore the long-term relationship between the Mediterranean Diet and body weight.[20] The trials evaluated the impact of the Mediterranean Diet on weight loss for 12 months or longer in overweight or obese subjects. The participants, though all overweight or obese at baseline, were screened for a range of comorbidities, including heart disease and type 2 diabetes. A total of 998 participants were included, ranging from 44 to 67 years of age with body mass indices of 29.7–33.5 kg/m^2. As with other systematic reviews and meta-analyses, the studies included in Mancini and colleague's research had a variety of definitions for the Mediterranean Diet. The prescribed diets varied based on fat content, calorie content, and focus on a "traditional" Mediterranean Diet or a "Mediterranean-style" Diet. Further, the control groups ranged from low-fat diets to low carbohydrate diets, and may or may not have also included calorie restriction. The studies followed their participants for a minimum of 12 months and up to as long as four years. To be included in the systematic review, studies that incorporated a physical activity recommendation or some type of nutrition counseling or education must have provided these aspects of intervention to both the treatment and control groups. In the end, long-term weight loss results varied widely. Some studies showed a significant difference in weight loss for the Mediterranean Diet group compared with a low-fat control group after just 12 months of follow-up. Other studies showed significant weight loss or change in body mass index in the Mediterranean Diet group compared with multiple controls (e.g., low fat and low carbohydrate diets), but only after one-and-a-half to two years of follow-up had elapsed. Many studies showed no significant change in body mass index after any length of follow-up. Nevertheless, the authors conclude a favorable outcome for the Mediterranean Diet when compared only with a low-fat control, but not with other diets (e.g., low carbohydrate, American Diabetic Association diet). Overall, they are unable to conclude that the Mediterranean Diet provides a weight loss advantage over other weight loss diets among overweight or obese participants.

The most recent analysis of data from the PREDIMED trial also assesses the effectiveness of a Mediterranean Diet to generate weight loss.[21] The multi-center trial with a parallel, randomized controlled design ran for five years among 7,447 participants. Study participants were middle-age and elderly (aged 55–80) Spanish men and women with type 2 diabetes or cardiovascular risk factors. As previously described, the study set out with a primary goal of assessing the impact of the Mediterranean Diet on cardiovascular health and was able to reinforce the positive findings of previous research on this topic. This most recent analysis aimed to tease out the effect of the Mediterranean Diet alone on weight loss, in the absence of calorie restriction or exercise recommendations. In the PREDIMED study design, participants were randomized to one of three study groups: Mediterranean Diet supplemented with olive oil, Mediterranean Diet supplemented with nuts, or a low-fat diet. Participants in all three groups received nutrition education from dietitians, though frequency and intensity of education varied between the treatment and control groups. All three groups received guidance on how many servings from each food group they should consume per day, which foods were recommended, and which foods should be avoided. None of the participants were placed on a calorie restriction nor provided any advice for recommended daily calorie intake. Similarly, there was no instruction or recommendation made with regard to exercise. After five years of follow-up, the research team found a significant reduction in body weight among participants following the Mediterranean Diet supplemented with olive oil when compared with the control group following the low-fat diet. The difference in reduction in body weight between the participants following the Mediterranean Diet supplemented with nuts and the control participants following the low-fat diet was not significant. The authors did find a significant reduction in central adiposity as measured by waist circumference in both the Mediterranean Diet groups (those participants supplemented with olive oil and those supplemented with nuts) when compared to the control group following the low-fat diet. The team concluded that the Mediterranean Diet can lead to successful weight loss compared to a standard, low-fat diet. Notably, these conclusions should be interpreted carefully since the study did not take into account calorie intake and expenditure. Hopefully, the forthcoming results from the PREDIMED-Plus trial—which is solely focused on overweight and obese subjects—will be able to shed additional light on the impact of the Mediterranean Diet on body weight specifically in this population.

TYPICAL RESULTS

At this time, there is insufficient evidence to support the Mediterranean Diet as an effective weight loss diet plan. This is due, in part, to the fact that the Mediterranean Diet was conceived through early observation in the 1950s of a diet and lifestyle practiced by individuals living along the Mediterranean Sea. The initial goal in assessing the health benefits of the Mediterranean Diet was not weight loss, but cardiovascular health and general longevity. And while organizations like Oldways Preservation Trust and the Fundación Dieta Mediterránea have created generally prescriptive food pyramids to guide patients who wish to follow the Mediterranean Diet, these recommendations are geared toward overall health and cardiovascular health, not toward weight loss.[10,11]

Further, discrepancies in the most recent research make it difficult to determine how patients' weight or body mass index may be positively impacted by the Mediterranean Diet. As previously noted, some studies show significant weight loss or change in body mass index with the Mediterranean Diet when compared to other more commonly used diets for weight loss such as low fat or low carbohydrate plans. Unfortunately, still other studies show no significant differences between the effects on body weight and/or body mass index of the Mediterranean Diet and other weight loss programs. The range of results can be attributed to the previously discussed lack of standardization in many aspects of the research, not the least of which is the definition of the Mediterranean Diet itself. Comparison against a wide range of control diets makes it difficult to pin down whether the Mediterranean Diet may create superior levels of weight loss than, for example, a low-fat diet or a low carbohydrate diet. Also, inconsistencies in including calorie restriction and physical activity recommendations in these studies make it difficult to interpret the results. It should also be noted that various lengths of follow-up—including some with quite short durations—in these studies may mean that longer term weight loss or simple avoidance of weight gain may not be captured by the data.

That said, some of the research conducted on the Mediterranean Diet in the last decade has shown some promising results with respect to weight loss despite these limitations. Recent studies hint at high levels of adherence to the Mediterranean Diet over time, so it is possible that, though initial weight loss results may not be as dramatic as with other diets, the Mediterranean Diet may be easier or more pleasurable for patients to comply with in the long term. Other studies have shown significantly reduced central adiposity or waist circumference with the Mediterranean Diet when compared with control diets, which can improve the patient's weight-related comorbidities.[21]

It should be reiterated that there have been several studies showing the clear reduction in cardiovascular disease risk associated with the Mediterranean Diet compared with other standards of care such as a low-fat diet. The results of these studies should not be minimized, and the Mediterranean Diet should be considered for patients whose health goals are broader than weight loss. Additionally, for patients whose health goals not only include weight loss but also improvement in type 2 diabetes or hypertension, the Mediterranean Diet should also be considered alongside alternatives like the Therapeutic Lifestyle Changes diet, the American Diabetes Association diet, low fat, or low carbohydrate diet options.

For some patients, it is possible that simply switching to the Mediterranean Diet alone may create lasting weight loss results. This may be due to the fact that the patient would have to cut back on certain food groups (e.g., red meat, sweets) that are found in abundance in the Western diet, and round out their eating habits with other foods that are more nutrient dense and lower in calories (e.g., fruits, vegetables, whole grains). Patients who desire weight loss may find increased satiety by switching to the Mediterranean Diet, due to the relative increased intake of lean proteins, fiber, and heart healthy fat. However, portion control for the higher calorie foods in this diet plan (i.e., nuts, olive oil, etc.) needs to be emphasized to patients.

In summary, it is crucial to reiterate that the Mediterranean Diet has never been a specific meal plan or regimen geared toward generating weight loss. Because of this, any given patient's weight loss experience may vary widely, and there is no such thing as a "typical" weight loss result when following the Mediterranean Diet. If weight loss is the desired primary goal of adopting the Mediterranean Diet, this decision should be carefully discussed with the patient's physician and a Registered Dietitian. It is important that patients recognize that simply shifting their eating habits to a Mediterranean Diet alone may not create weight loss. Education on calorie consumption, portion control, and lifestyle, especially physical activity, should be emphasized to patients.

PROS AND CONS

Pros

The Mediterranean Diet has a sizeable upside—it tastes great. Given the relatively high proportion of dietary fat included in the Mediterranean Diet, this is not surprising. Fat, primarily in the form of olive oil and nuts, helps carry fat-soluble flavor molecules, lends richness, and offers a pleasing mouth feel. Further, the Mediterranean Diet allows consumers to indulge in small portions of high-fat foods that might be considered verboten in other diets—nuts, cheese, and oil. In addition to fat, the Mediterranean Diet's reliance on the use of herbs and spices, onions, and garlic also leans toward intensely flavored food. A general focus on locally grown, seasonal produce also enhances flavor, as fruits and vegetables are picked and eaten at peak ripeness and maximum tastiness. Finally, the inclusion of alcohol—in moderation—allows for more flexibility for the inclusion of cultural norms, social occasions, and celebrations. In many ways, the importance of taste in the Mediterranean Diet can make it feel much more indulgent than the typical prescribed diet plan. This emphasis on flavor and feelings of indulgence may contribute to long-term adherence among weight loss patients, especially those who do not feel that they should be required to "give up" taste and enjoyment of foods in order to lose weight.

In addition to playing a role in the taste of the Mediterranean Diet, the relatively high dietary fat content also plays a crucial role in another key aspect of weight management: satiety. By slowing gastric emptying, heart healthy unsaturated fats like those found in olive oil, nuts, and seafood can help promote an improved feeling of satisfaction, even when portion sizes and calorie intake are moderated for weight loss. In weight management, lack of satiety can sabotage success by leading to unplanned snacking, grazing, or even binging. By including a moderate amount of dietary fat, the Mediterranean Diet may help encourage weight loss by avoiding excess calorie intake outside of structured meal and snack times. Fat is not the only factor promoting gratification in the Mediterranean Diet, though. The large volume of fruits and vegetables, as well as a focus on other plant foods—such as beans, legumes, and whole grains—results in a relatively high intake of dietary fiber. Dietary fiber helps promote fullness at meal times by expanding in the gut and triggering hormonal and neurological signals to the brain to indicate that the stomach is full.

The emphasis on dietary fiber and heart healthy fats has several other residual health benefits for devotees of the Mediterranean Diet, even if the primary goal of the diet is weight loss. High intake of dietary fiber from a plant-based diet like the Mediterranean Diet also helps promote gastrointestinal regularity, which may improve bloating and other gastrointestinal quality-of-life issues among patients. The high fiber intake of the Mediterranean Diet also helps to improve the lipid profile of patients by working to reduce serum cholesterol, and thus reduce their overall cardiovascular disease risk. Similarly, the Mediterranean Diet's focus on unsaturated fats—monounsaturated fats from olive oil and nuts, omega-3 poly-unsaturated fats from fish and nuts—as well as promotion of an active lifestyle also serves to improve the lipid profile. Monounsaturated fats have been shown to help lower low-density lipoprotein (LDL) cholesterol without impacting high-density lipoprotein (HDL) cholesterol, while omega-3 poly-unsaturated fats have been shown to both lower LDL cholesterol and possibly have a beneficial effect on HDL cholesterol levels.

The Mediterranean Diet further promotes overall health by promoting blood glucose control and insulin sensitivity. The Mediterranean Diet as described is very low in refined and added sugars. Though carbohydrate intake per the Mediterranean Diet is moderate—neither especially high nor especially low   most carbohydrate comes in the form of high fiber foods such as beans, legumes, and whole grains. The high fiber content of these foods reduces the effective impact of their consumption on blood sugar. In addition, intake of sweets is very limited, and dairy consumption—though recommended regularly or even daily—is advised in small portions. Perhaps because of the relatively high fiber nature of the Mediterranean Diet, or because of the low frequency with which sweets are consumed—or a combination of these factors—it seems as though the Mediterranean Diet can be useful in staving off the onset of type 2 diabetes. In a study published in 2014, researchers analyzing data from the PREDIMED trial were able to quantitatively show a positive impact of the Mediterranean Diet on incidence of type 2 diabetes among Spanish adults deemed at high risk for cardiovascular disease.[15] The team showed a statistically significant 30% reduction in risk for the development of type 2 diabetes among participants who adopted the Mediterranean Diet supplemented with either nuts or olive oil, compared with those who adopted a typical low-fat diet. Notably, these results were achieved with adoption of the Mediterranean Diet, but in the absence of calorie restriction.

As with most diets, the Mediterranean Diet acknowledges the important role of physical activity in maintaining health and promoting a healthy weight. But the Mediterranean Diet also recognizes another key aspect in overall well-being: social interaction, especially around food and eating. This unique aspect of the Mediterranean Diet can serve several purposes from a weight management perspective. As previously discussed, by taking time to enjoy social company along with the meal, for example, by engaging in conversation while dining—patients may be able to slow intake and better recognize physical and cognitive cues for fullness and satiety. Through mindful eating, patients may be able to increase enjoyment of foods, and possibly limit intake of snack foods. By reducing or eliminating mindless eating, and slowing intake of pleasurable foods, patients may be able to reduce calorie intake.

From a practical perspective, the Mediterranean Diet offers another key benefit for patients: flexibility. As the Mediterranean Diet pyramid suggests, no particular foods are "off-limits." Rather, even patients' favorite foods may be eaten in moderation or sparingly. This, of course, requires restraint on the part of the patient, and guidance, coaching, and support from the healthcare provider to reinforce healthy moderation and help modify more regular intake of, for example, meats and sweets. For some patients, though, knowing simply that no specific foods are included on a "do not eat" list may provide peace of mind and the motivation to continue with a diet, even when weight loss seems daunting. Similarly, knowing that favorite foods such as pasta may be included can also be a motivating factor for patients trying to lose weight. However, for patients without a sweet tooth, pescetarians already eschewing red meats and poultry, or those who prefer cheese and yogurt to cake and candy, the Mediterranean Diet may provide the appropriate amount of dietary flexibility to allow for both weight loss and enjoyment of food.

For weight management patients with spouses, families, or other living companions, the Mediterranean Diet may offer a mutually agreeable lifestyle that promotes health for all involved, and weight loss for those who desire. Holistically, the emphasis on flavorful foods, the lack of strict exclusions from the diet, and the focus on communal meals make the Mediterranean Diet a good choice for the entire household. Further, the plant-based nature of the diet can help keep the household food budget in check. Though the spirit of the Mediterranean Diet is rooted in locally grown, seasonably available produce, the "letter of the law" may easily be followed with frozen fruits and vegetables, inexpensive whole grains such as brown rice, and budget-friendly purchases like beans and legumes. Fish and seafood may be obtained inexpensively in the form of canned (packed in water) or preserved options, or frozen varieties as well. Herbs and spices may be procured in their dried form. Emphasis on seeking local farmer's markets which in many areas are offered all-year-round may be a plausible option for patients to purchase cost-effective fresh foods. More expensive animal products like meat and poultry can be used sparingly, keeping costs to a minimum. And processed and packaged foods, which may have low short term economic costs followed by high health costs for the whole family in the long term, can be avoided.

Cons

Conversely, some crucial components of the Mediterranean Diet can be expensive to obtain in parts of the world. Olive oil is often more expensive than other vegetable oils, though extra virgin olive oil specifically—the most expensive of the olive oils—is not necessary. Nuts and seeds can be pricey as well, although bulk purchases of these items can help to reduce cost. For patients who prefer to use only fresh products, the cost of abundant fruits and vegetables for an entire household can add up quickly, especially during winter months when they may not be locally available. And fresh, sustainably caught fish can indeed be quite costly. For lower income patients—especially those living in food deserts where supermarkets, farmer's markets, or other means of obtaining fresh groceries are not available—following the Mediterranean Diet may simply not be feasible. Similarly, in order to keep the cost of following the Mediterranean Diet in check, some cooking is required. Patients who do not like cooking, do not have time to cook, or do not have the skills to prepare food may not find the Mediterranean Diet compatible with their lifestyle. However, patients of certain means who enjoy eating outside the home regularly may be able to maintain the Mediterranean Diet by selecting restaurants with a focus on seasonal produce and seafood. It is important to acknowledge that restaurants may rely on saturated fats such as butter in their cooking, though, which is not aligned with the Mediterranean Diet. Similarly, patients who rely on fast foods, take out, and fast casual foods may find that the foods available, and their methods of preparation, do not align with the Mediterranean Diet.

Because the Mediterranean Diet does include regular use of some calorie dense foods—such as olive oil, nuts, legumes, and grains—portion control is an important consideration when using the diet for weight management. While patients may derive cardiovascular and other health benefits from switching to a more plant-based approach focused on unsaturated fats like the Mediterranean Diet, this switch alone will not necessarily create weight loss. In order to create the calorie deficit required for weight loss, patients must be educated about the appropriate portion sizes for these calorie dense foods. Further, patients and healthcare providers must frankly discuss the frequency with which foods such as meats and sweets will be consumed. For this purpose, use of the Mediterranean Diet pyramids as educational aids can be helpful, as they provide guidance for servings of these foods each day or week. While patients who struggle with portion control may find the relatively high intake of heart healthy fats and dietary fiber helpful with feelings of fullness and satiety, excessive intake of these fats, nuts, or grains may in fact lead to weight gain.

It is important to note that the Mediterranean Diet fails to address other issues in weight management. For example, the Mediterranean Diet does not explicitly take into account the way food is prepared beyond strongly suggesting the use of olive oil as the main source of fat. Neither the Oldways Preservation Trust pyramid nor the Fundación Dieta Mediterránea pyramid explicitly include guidance on intake of fried foods, baked goods, or sugar-sweetened beverages—all major sources of excess calories.[10,11] The spirit of the Mediterranean Diet is rooted in the consumption of minimally processed, simply prepared, mainly plant-based foods—but it is certainly possible to follow the "letter of the law" as described by the pyramids, while still continuing with consumption of high calorie fried foods such as fish and vegetables, and sugary drinks or pastry. As such, successful use of the Mediterranean Diet for weight loss depends on nutrition education and effective communication of the spirit of the Mediterranean pattern of eating.

IS THIS DIET RIGHT FOR YOUR PATIENTS?

The Mediterranean Diet can be a good fit for many types of patients wishing to improve their health and also possibly lose weight. Patients who struggle with satiety on other diets may find the extra fat and fiber in the Mediterranean Diet helpful. Those who already love fruits and vegetables may find the transition to a Mediterranean Diet easy to make. Similarly, the Mediterranean Diet can easily be adapted to suit a pescetarian, (ovo-lacto) vegetarian, or even vegan lifestyle. Patients who feel they are unable to give up pasta, bread, and other carbohydrates may be able to adapt more easily to the Mediterranean Diet. Conversely, patients who love red meat and poultry, or those for whom processed food is a matter-of-fact reality, may not readily take to the Mediterranean Diet. And as with any weight loss approach, the success of the Mediterranean Diet to create clinically significant and lasting weight changes depends mainly on the patient's willingness to make lifestyle modifications.

As previously mentioned, cooking can play an important role in successful transition to the Mediterranean Diet. Cooking one's own food offers added control over ingredients—for example, ensuring unsaturated fats like olive oil are used for cooking—and more careful attention to the composition of the meal with a proclivity toward plants and away from animal proteins. Patients who enjoy cooking or wish to do more of it may be more successful in adhering to the Mediterranean Diet. For those who wish to learn how to cook or to hone their existing skills with an emphasis on the Mediterranean Diet, many cookbooks and cooking classes exist. However, for patients who also enjoy venturing outside the home to eat, the Mediterranean Diet can also accommodate restaurant foods when the appropriate establishments are selected for dining. Conversely, patients who—for reasons of necessity or otherwise—rely on packaged or processed foods, fast foods, or other convenience foods may not feasibly be able to follow the Mediterranean Diet for weight loss. In other words, it would be difficult to adhere to the spirit and the letter of the Mediterranean Diet solely from a convenience store or fast food restaurant.

Similarly, consideration of a patient's financial situation and ability to procure groceries is an important component of determining whether or not a patient might adhere to the Mediterranean Diet. In order to follow the diet as directed, patients will need access to markets (supermarkets or farmer's/open air markets) with produce (fresh or frozen), whole grains, seafood, and dairy (preferably low fat), with occasional ventures into the meat and poultry aisle. Also, patients will need access to appropriate storage at home (e.g., refrigeration and/or freezer). Ideally, patients will also need the financial ability and accessibility to obtain olive oil and other sources of unsaturated fats including nuts and oily fish.

As several studies have demonstrated, the Mediterranean Diet is an appropriate eating pattern for patients who wish to reduce their cardiovascular disease risk. Patients with a personal or family history of cardiovascular disease, or even hyperlipidemia, might consider the Mediterranean Diet for its health benefits alone, weight loss goals aside. Similarly, patients who currently have type 2 diabetes, are pre-diabetic, or have a high risk for type 2 diabetes—due to family history or other comorbidities—might also consider the Mediterranean Diet pattern for improved blood glucose control, and to reduce their own increased risk for cardiovascular disease. Additional studies have begun to point to the health benefits of the Mediterranean Diet in the prevention of various types of cancer, for cognitive decline associated with aging, and even possibly longevity.[6,7,22,23] Thus, for patients for whom overall health is the primary goal—and weight loss is a secondary outcome—the Mediterranean Diet may be a suitable choice.

Ultimately, the Mediterranean Diet is a diet for people who love the types of food the diet accommodates. It offers the freedom to eat foods that might otherwise be "forbidden" on other diets—such as pasta or cheese—and to drink alcohol in moderation. However, it is crucial that patients do not view a license to eat pasta, consume cheese, and drink alcohol as a sanction to consume large quantities of these foods or beverages. The Physician and Registered Dietitian play an important role in ensuring that any patient using the Mediterranean Diet for weight loss is able to understand the importance of portion control and moderation. It may be necessary to provide patients with a calorie prescription to guide their use of the Mediterranean Diet for weight management. Similarly, it might be helpful to have patients track their intake using a food log or food tracking smartphone application as an educational tool to learn about calorie consumption, portion control, and overall dietary habits. Finally, it may be important to involve an Exercise Physiologist or Certified Personal Trainer to incorporate daily physical activity per the Mediterranean Diet lifestyle.

REFERENCES

1. Seven Countries Study | The first study to relate diet with cardiovascular disease. The Seven Countries Study (SCS for short) is the first major study to look at dietary components and patterns and lifestyle as risk factors for cardiovascular disease, over multiple countries and extended periods of time. Seven Countries Study | The first study to relate diet with cardiovascular disease. http://www.sevencountriesstudy.com/ (accessed August 14, 2016).
2. Keys AB. *How to Eat Well and Stay Well the Mediterranean Way.* 1st edition. Garden City, NY: Doubleday; 1975.
3. Kushi LH, Lenart EB, Willett WC. Health implications of Mediterranean diets in light of contemporary knowledge. 1. Plant foods and dairy products. *Am J Clin Nutr* 1995;61(6 Suppl):1407S–15S.
4. Kushi LH, Lenart EB, Willett WC. Health implications of Mediterranean diets in light of contemporary knowledge. 2. Meat, wine, fats, and oils. *Am J Clin Nutr* 1995;61(6 Suppl):1416S–27S.
5. Fung TT, Hu FB, McCullough ML, Newby PK, Willett WC, Holmes MD. Diet quality is associated with the risk of estrogen receptor-negative breast cancer in postmenopausal women. *J Nutr* 2006;136(2):466–72.
6. Fung TT, McCullough ML, Newby PK. et al. Diet-quality scores and plasma concentrations of markers of inflammation and endothelial dysfunction. *Am J Clin Nutr* 2005;82(1):163–73.
7. Samieri C, Sun Q, Townsend MK. et al. The association between dietary patterns at midlife and health in aging: An observational study. *Ann Intern Med* 2013;159(9):584–91. doi:10.7326/0003-4819-159-9-201311050-00004.
8. De Lorgeril M, Salen P, Martin JL, Monjaud I, Delaye J, Mamelle N. Mediterranean diet, traditional risk factors, and the rate of cardiovascular complications after myocardial infarction: Final report of the Lyon Diet Heart Study. *Circulation* 1999;99(6):779–85.
9. Willett WC, Sacks F, Trichopoulou A. et al. Mediterranean diet pyramid: A cultural model for healthy eating. *Am J Clin Nutr* 1995;61(6 Suppl):1402S–6S.
10. Mediterranean Diet. Oldways. http://oldwayspt.org/traditional-diets/mediterranean-diet (accessed August 14, 2016).
11. Mediterranean Diet. *Fund Dieta Mediterr.* http://dietamediterranea.com/en/ (accessed August 14, 2016).
12. Mediterranean diet-intangible heritage-Culture Sector-UNESCO. http://www.unesco.org/culture/ich/en/RL/mediterranean-diet-00884 (accessed August 12, 2016).

13. Predimed.es - Home. http://www.predimed.es/ (accessed August 12, 2016).
14. Estruch R, Ros E, Salas-Salvadó J. et al. Primary prevention of cardiovascular disease with a Mediterranean diet. *N Engl J Med* 2013;368(14):1279–90. doi:10.1056/NEJMoa1200303.
15. Martínez-González MA, Estruch R, Corella D, Ros E, Salas-Salvadó J. Prevention of diabetes with Mediterranean diets. *Ann Intern Med* 2014;161(2):157–8. doi:10.7326/L14-5014-2.
16. PREDIMED PLUS. http://predimedplus.com/ (accessed August 15, 2016).
17. Buckland G, Bach A, Serra-Majem L. Obesity and the Mediterranean diet: A systematic review of observational and intervention studies. *Obes Rev* 2008;9(6):582–93. doi:10.1111/j.1467-789X.2008.00503.x.
18. Esposito K, Kastorini C-M, Panagiotakos DB, Giugliano D. Mediterranean diet and weight loss: Meta-analysis of randomized controlled trials. *Metab Syndr Relat Disord* 2010;9(1):1–12. doi:10.1089/met.2010.0031.
19. Gomez-Huelgas R, Jansen-Chaparro S, Baca-Osorio AJ, Mancera-Romero J, Tinahones FJ, Bernal-López MR. Effects of a long-term lifestyle intervention program with Mediterranean diet and exercise for the management of patients with metabolic syndrome in a primary care setting. *Eur J Intern Med* 2015;26(5):317–23. doi:10.1016/j.ejim.2015.04.007.
20. Mancini JG, Filion KB, Atallah R, Eisenberg MJ. Systematic review of the Mediterranean diet for long-term weight loss. *Am J Med* 2016;129(4):407–415.e4. doi:10.1016/j.amjmed.2015.11.028.
21. Estruch R, Martínez-González MA, Corella D. et al. Effect of a high-fat Mediterranean diet on bodyweight and waist circumference: A prespecified secondary outcomes analysis of the PREDIMED randomised controlled trial. *Lancet Diabetes Endocrinol* June 2016;4(8):666–76. doi:10.1016/S2213-8587(16)30085-7.
22. Hardman RJ, Kennedy G, Macpherson H, Scholey AB, Pipingas A. Adherence to a Mediterranean-style diet and effects on cognition in adults: A qualitative evaluation and systematic review of longitudinal and prospective trials. *Front Nutr* 2016;3:22. doi:10.3389/fnut.2016.00022.
23. García-Calzón S, Martínez-González MA, Razquin C. et al. Mediterranean diet and telomere length in high cardiovascular risk subjects from the PREDIMED-NAVARRA study. *Clin Nutr Edinb Scotl* April 2016. doi:10.1016/j.clnu.2016.03.013.

5 The Paleo Diet

Laura Andromalos

CONTENTS

OVERVIEW

If you have not yet heard of the Paleo Diet, you are in the minority. "Paleo" was the most searched diet-related term on Google in 2014.[1] It has inspired multiple magazines, podcasts, cookbooks, and cooking blogs and it has even led to the creation of strictly Paleo restaurants.[2] While the Paleo Diet craze is relatively recent, the concept of Paleolithic nutrition as a diet model has been around for over 40 years.

Its earliest roots can be traced back to 1975 when gastroenterologist Walter Voegtlin published *The Stone Age Diet*.[3] In his book, he writes: "The evidence is incontestable that Man's foods still should be those he naturally selected and even today digests with greatest ease—protein and fat with little or no carbohydrate."[3] The concept did not seem to catch on because it was another 10 years until it was introduced to the academic community and Voegtlin's work was not cited.[4]

S. Boyd Eaton and Melvin Konner formalized the concept of evolutionary nutrition in their 1985 article, Paleolithic nutrition, in the *New England Journal of Medicine*.[4] They proposed that modern humans are genetically programmed for a pre-agricultural diet, or a hunter-gatherer diet, because the genome has not evolved as quickly as the human diet.[4] Therefore, "diseases of civilization," coronary heart disease, hypertension, diabetes, and some types of cancer are a result of humans adopting a diet for which they are not appropriately evolved.[4] This is known as the evolutionary discordance hypothesis.

The Agricultural Revolution, which began about 10,000 years ago, is the period in which many humans discontinued the hunter-gatherer lifestyle and diet and began farming.[4] Although there were multiple hunter-gatherer diet compositions which were dependent upon geography, Eaton and Konner estimated that an average Paleolithic hunter-gatherer consumed 35% calories from protein, 45% from carbohydrates, and 21% from fat with a diet breakdown of 65% vegetation and 35% meat.[4] Carbohydrate sources included wild fruits and vegetables as well as roots, beans, tubers, and small amounts of grains.[4] Of note, this is significantly different from Voegtlin's proposal of a diet with little or no carbohydrate.[3] For those humans who adapted to farming, diets shifted from approximately 65% vegetation to 90% vegetation with a marked decrease in protein intake.[4] Eaton and Konner cite anthropological studies which demonstrate that human skeletons became shorter and showed manifestations of suboptimal nutrition in the generations immediately following the beginning of the Agricultural Revolution.[4] While their paper piqued interest in the academic community, the concept did not yet attract attention in the public.

About 10 years later, Loren Cordain began collaborating with Eaton on Paleolithic nutrition research.[5] As a professor in the Department of Health and Exercise Science at Colorado State University, Cordain's research was on the impact of diet on athletic performance and he became interested in Eaton's work.[5] In 2002, Cordain published the first iteration of The Paleo Diet.[6] While it was well-received in its first few years, it did not gain national exposure.[7] In 2010, the book was fully revised and caught fire among the public; Cordain attributes this surge in popularity to the development of internet culture which facilitates sharing of and searching for nutrition information.[7]

The Paleo Diet has also generated critical responses. Anthropological studies have demonstrated that starchy vegetation did play a role in the diets of many hunter-gatherers.[8-10] Interestingly, Eaton and Konner's original paper acknowledged this, but these foods were excluded from Cordain's Paleo Diet.[4,7] Other criticisms stem from the evolutionary nutrition concept that the human genome has not adapted in the past 10,000 years; lactose tolerance in adults is one example of an adaptation that has occurred during that time period.[11] Regardless of these criticisms, the Paleo Diet has become a popular health food trend in our society.

The popularity of evolutionary nutrition has generated several iterations of Paleolithic and caveman diets which have varying rules. Some involve intermittent fasting and others promote the consumption of any type of meat regardless of its fat content.[12-14] It is likely that many people who believe they are following the Paleo Diet have never read Cordain's book and are receiving their information from family, friends, gyms, or the internet. This chapter will not include reviews of all variations of a Paleolithic or caveman diet but only The Paleo Diet published in 2010 by Cordain.

HOW THE DIET WORKS

The Paleo Diet attempts to apply concepts from evolutionary nutrition theories into a modern diet. There is no calorie-counting and little reliance on portion control. Rather, the Paleo Diet entails lists of foods to be eaten or avoided as well as meal plan suggestions.

Cordain outlines six "ground rules" for the Paleo Diet, which will be expanded on in this chapter:[7]

1. All the lean meats, fish, and seafood you can eat
2. All the fruits and non-starchy vegetables you can eat
3. No cereals
4. No legumes
5. No dairy products
6. No processed foods

There is very little focus on calories and portions because the protein and fiber content of the diet are expected to provide satiety and naturally decrease intake, unless a person is eating for non-hunger reasons. The foods that are encouraged at every meal are lean animal foods, fruits, and vegetables.[7]

Lean Animal Foods: Dieters are advised to get just over half their daily calories from animal foods but they should be from lean sources. The Paleo Diet book provides a list of lean meats for guidance. Eggs should be limited to six to twelve per week due to the percent of calories from fat and ideally should be from free-range hens that are fed omega-3 enriched diets.

Fruits: For the most part, fresh fruits can be eaten without restriction. Cordain recommends that people who have obesity be more mindful of their total fruit consumption and that people with metabolic syndrome avoid "high-sugar fruits" such as grapes, bananas, cherries, and mangos. Dried fruit should be restricted to no more than 2 ounces daily, especially for those trying to lose weight.

Vegetables: Non-starchy vegetables can be eaten without restriction but high-carbohydrate vegetables, such as potatoes, are restricted.

In addition to these meal components, foods containing unsaturated fats should be consumed in moderation. Cordain describes the Paleo Diet as a "bad fat-free diet," as opposed to a fat-free diet.[7] Fat-rich foods included in the diet are nuts, avocados, seeds, and oils (flaxseed, olive, walnut, or avocado). The recommendation of moderation is most important for those who are trying to lose weight. In the context of weight loss, Cordain recommends limiting consumption to 4 ounces of nuts and 4 tablespoons of oil daily.[7]

Water is the primary beverage on the Paleo Diet. However, there are some other beverages that can be included in moderation. For those who currently drink alcohol, Cordain recommends limiting consumption to one 12-oz serving beer, two 4-oz servings wine, or one 4-oz serving of spirits daily. Any beverage containing artificial sweeteners should be limited to moderate consumption. Coffee and tea should be limited as well due to potential health problems associated with excess caffeine. Beverages that contain sugar, whether natural or added, are to be avoided.

Vitamin and mineral supplements can be taken as needed. While Cordain presents a nutrient analysis of a day on the Paleo Diet that exceeds the Recommended Dietary Allowances (RDAs) in most categories of micronutrients, he also acknowledges that supplements may be required for some people. For people who are not able to achieve adequate sun exposure for vitamin D production, he suggests supplementing up to 2000 IU vitamin D daily. Due to the presence of toxic substances that were not present in the Paleolithic environment, Cordain suggests supplementing some antioxidants beyond the levels achieved by the diet based on studies suggesting improved immune function and protection against cancer.[7] These include daily doses of 200–400 IU vitamin E, 500–1000 milligrams vitamin C, and 200–400 micrograms selenium. Last, he suggests fish oil capsules for those who are not including fish in their diet. His recommendation is 1–2 grams of eicosapentaenoic acid (EPA) and docosahexaenoic acid (DHA) daily to decrease the risk of cancer and heart disease.[7]

Lean protein, fruits, and vegetables are the mainstay of many popular diets. What sets the Paleo Diet apart from these other diets is the list of foods to be avoided. The rationale for avoiding these foods is their lack of presence in our ancestors' hunter-gatherer diets.[7] Cordain explains that a dieter does not have to banish these foods from their diet forever.[7] Weaning off these foods over time, whether it takes days, weeks, or months, is a reasonable approach as well. However, the following foods should ultimately be avoided while on the Paleo Diet:

- Any dairy products
- Grains, including barley, corn, millet, oats, rice, rye, sorghum, wheat, and wild rice
- Grain-like seeds, including amaranth, buckwheat, and quinoa
- Legumes, including peanuts and soy
- Starchy vegetables, including tubers, cassava root, manioc, potatoes, sweet potatoes, tapioca, and yams
- Salt-containing foods, including condiments, salted spices, pickled foods, and processed meats
- Fatty meats
- Sweetened beverages and fruit juice
- Added sugars

After understanding which foods and beverages to eat and to avoid, the next step is to decide how closely one would like to follow the Paleo Diet.

There are three levels of adherence to the Paleo Diet:

- Level I: Entry Level with three Open Meals per week
- Level II: Maintenance Level with two Open Meals per week
- Level III: Maximal Weight Loss Level with one Open Meal per week

The difference between the levels is the allowed number of "Open Meals," which are meals that do not follow the Paleo Diet rules (i.e., include foods from the avoid list). The Open Meals are intended to provide flexibility and make the diet sustainable in the long term. However, Open Meals should be limited to one per day and should not be considered an opportunity to overindulge in forbidden foods.

Level I is based on the 85–15 rule; 85% of food choices adhere to the Paleo Diet rules and 15% do not. Based on a person who is consuming 20 meals per week, 15% or three of the meals are Open Meals that can include foods from the avoid list. In addition to these Open Meals, a person in Level I has the flexibility to include some "transitional" foods that do not quite meet the Paleo Diet rules but are intended to help people move in the direction of allowed foods. Examples of these would be low-fat salad dressings which do contain sugar and salt but are low in fat or condiments such as mustard, hot sauce, and prepared salsa. Of note, the only ketchup allowed on the Paleo Diet, even in Level I, is a recipe for Paleo ketchup, which is lower in salt and sugar than commercial ketchups. Level II is considered a maintenance level. It should not include transitional foods, except during an Open Meal. Two Open Meals are allowed per week at this level of adherence. Level III is intended for the person who wants to receive the maximal health benefits from the Paleo Diet or for people with obesity or severe chronic disease.

It is important to note that a person does not necessarily progress through the levels. Cordain suggests that a beginner adhere to Level I for two to four weeks before advancing to Level II or III. However, a person does not have to advance to higher levels if one is happy with the results at Level I. Many people will be satisfied at Levels I or II and never feel the need to progress to Level III.

Snacks are allowed between meals as needed and a snack list is provided in the Paleo Diet book. Snacks composition follows the same rules as meal composition. They are comprised of lean animal foods, fruits, and non-starchy vegetables. Additionally, they may contain nuts, seeds, or avocado and do not include any foods/beverages from the avoid list.

CURRENT RESEARCH

In his book, Cordain emphasizes the impact of the Paleo Diet on diseases related to metabolic syndrome and insulin resistance, including type 2 diabetes, heart disease, hypertension, dyslipidemia, obesity, polycystic ovarian syndrome, myopia, acne, and breast, prostate, and colon cancers.[7] Most of the published literature on Paleolithic diets has focused on metabolic syndrome and insulin resistance and will be discussed in this section.

In addition, Cordain writes that the Paleo Diet can improve diseases of acid-base balance and excess sodium, digestive diseases, inflammatory diseases, autoimmune diseases, psychological disorders, and skin cancers.[7] There are aspects of the Paleo Diet that have been linked to improvements in some of these conditions. For example, the foods of the Paleo Diet have low potential renal acid load (PRAL) and this type of alkaline diet has been found to have a range of potential health benefits.[15] An alkaline diet is rich in fruits and vegetables, which improves the potassium to sodium ratio in the body; this has beneficial implications for bone status, muscle wasting, and chronic disease including hypertension and strokes.[15] Some research suggests that dairy and grains can worsen symptoms in people with irritable bowel disease (IBD).[16] Since these food groups are excluded in the Paleo Diet, it could be argued that the diet improves health status in people with digestive disease. On the other hand, there is also research to suggest that while diets high in fiber, fruits, and vegetables decrease risk for developing IBD, a diet high in meat increases risk.[17] The diet is high in omega-3 fatty acids, which have been suggested to have anti-inflammatory properties that can delay the development of atherosclerosis.[18] However, the Paleo Diet as a whole has not been studied in the specific context of these diseases.

The research that has been published using a Paleolithic diet intervention is reviewed below. The Paleolithic diets used in these studies were explained in various levels of detail and sometimes divert from each other in terms of allowed and not allowed foods and beverages. Generally, all diets eliminated dairy products, cereals/grains, legumes, and added sugars. Beyond that, there was variation in terms of some foods and beverages such as eggs, alcohol, and starchy vegetables. These variations will be noted in the description of each study.

In 2007, Lindeberg and colleagues published results from a 12-week diet intervention study with 29 men that had ischemic heart disease and either impaired glucose tolerance or type 2 diabetes.[19] Fourteen participants (average age 65 years) were randomized to a Paleolithic diet and 15 (average age 57 years) to a Consensus diet, which was based on a Mediterranean Diet. The groups had comparable rates of impaired glucose tolerance and type 2 diabetes. The Paleolithic diet followed the above guidelines and contained limited amounts of the following foods: eggs (one or fewer per day), nuts (ideally walnuts due to omega-3 fatty acid content), potatoes (two or fewer per day), rapeseed or olive oil (one or fewer tablespoons per day), and wine (one or fewer glasses per day). Beer was not allowed. No advice was given regarding the proportion of animal versus plant foods in the diet. Notable differences between the diet interventions were the inclusion of whole grains, legumes, and low-fat dairy in the Consensus diet. After 12 weeks of diet intervention, the two groups were comparable in terms of weight loss, but the Paleolithic diet group had a significantly greater decrease in waist circumference compared to the Consensus diet group (5.6 cm versus 2.9 cm; p = 0.03). Additionally, the Paleolithic diet group had a marked improvement in plasma glucose with a decrease of 26% over the 12 weeks as opposed to 7% in the Consensus diet group. This change was independent of weight loss and waist circumference. The authors concluded that a Paleolithic diet could effectively improve glucose tolerance independent of waist circumference.[19]

Lindeberg and colleagues also published results from a randomized cross-over diet study with 13 adult men and women with type 2 diabetes (average age 64 years).[20] Most participants were taking oral medications for diabetes; average duration of diabetes was nine years and average HbA1c was 6.6%. Participants were randomized to either a Paleolithic diet (as described above) or a "diabetes diet." The diabetes diet included non-starchy and starchy vegetables, whole grains, and fruits, with an emphasis on unsaturated fat and overall decrease in total fat and a recommended salt intake of less than 6 grams/day. Participants were provided with written advice on their diet assignment along with recipes. Each diet intervention lasted three months. Six weeks into each diet intervention, diet adherence was monitored through a four-day food record that included the weight of each food consumed. Although participants were not told to restrict food intake, the reported energy intake was lower on the Paleolithic diet compared to the diabetes diet, which resulted in greater weight loss (delta of 3 kg; p = 0.01) and reduction in waist circumference (delta of 4 cm; p = 0.02) in the Paleolithic diet. The Paleolithic diet resulted in better glycemic control as evidenced by a delta of 0.4% for HbA1C levels (p = 0.02). In addition, the Paleolithic diet facilitated significantly greater improvements in several cardiometabolic risk factors including triglycerides (delta of 0.4 mmol/L; p = 0.003), diastolic blood pressure (delta of 4 mm Hg; p = 0.03), and high-density lipoprotein (HDL) cholesterol (delta of 0.08 mmol/L; p = 0.03). The researchers concluded that a 3-month Paleolithic diet intervention improved glycemic control and cardiometabolic risk factors compared to a diabetes diet.[20]

A second paper from this study was published in 2013 to report on the perceived satiety of the diet interventions.[21] Participants reported equal satiety on both diets; however, since they had consumed fewer calories on the Paleolithic diet, the satiety quotient was greater for energy per meal on the Paleolithic diet versus the diabetes diet. Based on qualitative data in response to open-ended questions about the two diets, the Paleolithic diet was considered helpful for weight loss but more difficult to adhere to when compared with the diabetes diet.[21]

Osterdahl and colleagues published the outcomes of a 3-week Paleolithic diet intervention on cardiovascular risk factors in 14 healthy adult men and women ages 20–40 years.[22] The Paleolithic diet allowed unlimited amounts of flaxseed or rape-seed oil for salad dressing and unlimited amounts of coffee and tea. Restricted foods included dry fruit (two times per week), salted seafood, high-fat meat, cured meat (one time each per week), honey (one time per week), and potatoes (two per day). Alcohol and eggs were not mentioned. Due to a computer error, they were only able to analyze the normal and intervention diets of six participants. From the records of those six participants, favorable changes resulting from the Paleolithic diet included a decrease in saturated fat intake, increased intake of vitamins C and E, and an increase in the potassium to sodium ratio. An unfavorable change was decreased average intake of calcium from 851 to 395 mg daily. All 14 patients had decreases in weight (2.3 kg; $p = 0.000$), waist circumference (1.5 cm; $p = 0.001$), and systolic blood pressure (3 mm Hg; $p = 0.03$). Although the study was underpowered, the researchers concluded that a short-term Paleolithic diet can have some favorable effects on nutrient intake.[22]

In 2009, Frassetto and colleagues published results from a 10-day Paleolithic diet intervention in nine healthy adult men and women (average age 38 years).[23] Participants were given one week of ramp up diets to prepare their bodies for the increased potassium and fiber load. Eggs, honey, and canola oil were included in the diet intervention, but alcohol was not mentioned. All meals and snacks were prepared in the research center; participants ate one meal in the research center and brought the remaining meals and snacks home. The diet was modified to prevent weight loss based on daily weights of the participants. After the diet intervention, participants had reduction in mean arterial pressure (3.1 mm Hg; $p = 0.01$), total cholesterol (0.7 mmol/L; $p = 0.007$), low-density lipoprotein (LDL) cholesterol (0.7 mmol/L; $p = 0.003$), and triglycerides (0.3 mmol/L; $p = 0.01$) when compared to measures from their baseline diet. The researchers concluded that a Paleolithic diet can improve some metabolic and physiologic metrics independent of weight loss.[23]

Boers and colleagues published a randomized controlled single-blind trial comparing the outcomes of a 2-week Paleolithic diet to an isoenergic reference diet based on the guidelines of the Dutch Health Council.[24] Participants were 32 adult men and women with at least two characteristics of metabolic syndrome; 18 participants were in the Paleolithic diet group (average age 52 years) and 16 were in the reference diet group (average age 55.4 years). The Paleolithic diet included eggs, root vegetables, and up to two cups of black coffee or tea daily. Notable differences between the diet interventions were inclusion of whole grains and low-fat dairy in the reference diet. At the end of the 2-week diet intervention, participants in the Paleolithic diet group had greater reductions in diastolic blood pressure (delta of 5.2 mm Hg;

p = 0.04), total cholesterol (delta of 0.5 mmol/L; p = 0.04), and triglycerides (delta 0.9 mmol/L; p = 0.00) than in the reference diet group. Although measures were taken to keep weight stable, participants in both groups lost weight, with those in the Paleolithic diet group losing 1.3 kg more than those in the reference diet group (p = 0.01). Upon analysis, the positive health effects were independent of the unintended weight loss. Additional outcomes of intestinal permeability, inflammation, and cortisol were not impacted by the diet intervention. The researchers concluded that a 2-week Paleolithic diet improved several cardiovascular risk factors in participants with metabolic syndrome compared to a reference healthy diet.[24]

In 2014, Whalen and colleagues published a paper regarding the risk of colorectal polyps based on diet history.[25] They used data from a previous case-controlled research program that tracked the incidence of colorectal polyps. Using a 12-month food frequency questionnaire, which had been completed by each participant in the previous research program, Whalen and colleagues scored the reported intake based on how well it matched the principles of either a Mediterranean or Paleolithic diet pattern and sorted the scores into quintiles. Based on their analysis, they concluded that greater adherence to either a Paleolithic or a Mediterranean Diet was associated with lower risk of colorectal adenomas when compared to a traditional Western diet.[25]

Mellberg and colleagues published results from a 24-month Paleolithic diet intervention study. They randomized 70 post-menopausal women with obesity to either an *ad libitum* Paleolithic diet (average age 59.5 years) or a diet based on the Nordic Nutrition Recommendations (NNR) (average age 60.3 years) for 24 months.[26] The Paleolithic diet targeted 30% calories from protein, 40% from fat, and 30% from carbohydrates and included eggs. In the NNR diet, participants aimed for 15% calories from protein, 25%–30% from fat, and 55%–60% from carbohydrates with an emphasis on low-fat dairy foods and high-fiber foods. Participants attended 12 group sessions over the 24-month period, which involved cooking classes, behavioral change therapies, and nutrition advice provided by trained study dietitians. Dietary adherence was monitored through 4-day self-reports monthly for the first six months and every three months thereafter. After six months of the intervention, participants in the Paleolithic diet group had significantly greater fat and weight loss than those in the NNR diet group; however, at the 24-month mark, the difference between the diet groups was not sustained. Reductions in fat mass, weight, and waist circumference were seen in both groups at the 24-month mark. The only significant difference between the groups at the 24-month mark was a greater decrease in triglycerides in the Paleolithic diet group versus the NNR diet group (0.23 mmol/L versus 0.1 mmol/L; p = 0.04). At the end of the study period, 77% of participants remained in the Paleo Diet group versus 63% in the NNR diet group. Based on urinary nitrogen, the researchers determined that participants in the Paleolithic diet group struggled to achieve the protein intake goal of 30% energy, which suggests that diet components other than protein intake contribute to the beneficial effects of a Paleolithic diet.[26]

Smith and colleagues in 2014 studied the impact of a 10-week *ad libitum* Paleolithic diet on the blood lipid profiles of 44 healthy and active adult men and women (average age of 33.5 years for males and 33.2 years for females).[27] Participants were given information regarding the Paleolithic diet described by Eaton and Konner but were not given macronutrient recommendations or guidelines for proportion of animal versus plant foods. In addition to the diet intervention, they participated in a high-intensity CrossFit-based circuit training program. The exercise was not controlled; frequency was described as "regularly" and no details were provided regarding duration. At the end of the 10-week intervention, body weight (80.7–77.5 kg; P < 0.01) and fat (24.3%–20.7%; P < 0.05) decreased significantly while LDL cholesterol (93.1–105.6 mg/dL; P < 0.01) and total cholesterol (168.8–178.9 mg/dL; P < 0.05) increased significantly. The authors concluded that an *ad libitum* unrestricted Paleolithic diet can have a negative impact on blood lipid profiles in healthy, active adults.[27]

Masharani and colleagues published an outpatient, metabolically controlled, 2-week diet study in adults with type 2 diabetes in 2015.[28] Participants were randomized to either a Paleolithic diet or an American Diabetes Association (ADA) diet. The Paleolithic diet included honey but excluded potatoes and products containing potassium chloride. The ADA diet contained low-fat dairy, whole grains, legumes, and about 4100 mg sodium daily. There were 14 participants in the Paleolithic diet group (average age 58 years with average HbA1C 7.3%) and 10 in the ADA diet group (average age 56 years with average HbA1C 7.0%). The majority of participants were on oral medications for diabetes; this did not change during the study period. Participants in the Paleolithic diet group were ramped up for a week to allow their bodies to adjust to the increased fiber and potassium load of the diet due to the increased intake of fruits and vegetables. After the intervention, weight loss was similar in both diet groups (2.4 kg in Paleolithic diet versus 2.1 kg in ADA diet). In terms of lipids, participants in the Paleolithic diet group had statistically significant reductions in total cholesterol (26 mg/dL; p = 0.003), HDL cholesterol (8 mg/dL; p = 0.001) and LDL cholesterol (15 mg/dL; p = 0.02), whereas participants in the ADA diet group had only significant reductions in HDL cholesterol (6 mg/dL; p = 0.03). Both groups had improvements in insulin sensitivity that was independent of weight loss; the difference was statistically significant for the Paleolithic diet group but not for the ADA diet group. Within the Paleolithic diet group, participants who were the most insulin resistant at baseline had the greatest improvements. The researchers concluded that even a short-term Paleolithic diet can improve glucose control and lipid panels in people with type 2 diabetes compared to a conventional diabetes diet.[28]

Bligh and colleagues investigated the acute impact of Paleolithic diet meals on gut hormones and appetite using a randomized, cross-over trial.[29] Study participants were healthy adult men (average age 27.5 years). The researchers developed three meals:

- REF: Reference meal based on World Health Organization guidelines with 383 calories, 60% calories from carbohydrates, 25% from fat, 15% from protein; contained rice, mango, carrots, salmon, and olive oil
- PAL1: Paleolithic meal with 556 calories, 43% calories from carbohydrates, 28% from fat, 29% from protein (estimated macronutrient percentages consumed by hunter-gatherers); contained variety of non-starchy vegetables and fruits, haddock and salmon, nuts, capers, and flaxseed oil
- PAL2: Paleolithic meal with the same ingredients as PAL1 but matched to the caloric content and macronutrient percentages of the reference diet

Each meal was consumed in the research lab on three separate occasions (1 meal on each occasion) with a 2-week break between each meal. Glucagon-like peptide 1 (GLP-1) and peptide YY (PYY) concentrations were significantly increased after both PAL1 and PAL2 compared to REF while glucose-dependent insulinotropic peptide GIP concentrations were significantly suppressed. These biomarkers indicate increased satiety with the PAL1 and PAL2 meals as compared to the REF meal. Additionally, satiation, measured through electronic visual analog scale, was reported at significantly higher levels for PAL1 and PAL2 versus REF. There was no significant difference in glucose and insulin levels between the three meals. Since PAL2 was lower in calories than PAL1 but had the same impact on anorectic hormones and satiety, the researchers suggested this meal composition could be effective for weight control.[29]

TYPICAL RESULTS

This section will summarize the results from the studies discussed above. Please note, the majority of the studies investigating Paleolithic diets are small with homogenous populations so the data regarding expected results must be interpreted with caution.

ANTHROPOMETRICS

Paleolithic diets have been effective at promoting weight loss in the short-term, even when the weight loss is unintentional.[22,24,28] Since they are low-carbohydrate diets, most people will initially lose water weight. Beyond that, weight loss could vary greatly since the Paleo Diet does not have a calorie recommendation.[7] Based on the research studies discussed in the previous section, study participants lost at least 2%–3.5% of total body weight two to three weeks after starting the diet.[22,24,28] After 10–12 weeks, participants had lost 4%–6% of total body weight.[19,27] Only one study reported on weight loss after one to two years of a Paleolithic diet intervention; their participants had lost a total of 10% body weight at one year but regained weight for a total of 7% body weight lost at two years.[26]

Several of the studies measured waist circumference. Based on this data, participants with normal body mass index (BMI) as well as with overweight and obesity had reduction in waist circumference by 2%–2.7% after two to three weeks of diet intervention and a reduction of 5.2%–5.3% after 12 weeks of intervention.[19,20,22,24] The long-term study reported a 10% reduction in waist circumference after one year of intervention; however, after two years of intervention, the total reduction in waist circumference was only 3.7%.[26]

LIPID PANEL LEVELS

Most of the studies that included lipid panel levels reported favorable changes in response to short-term Paleolithic diets.[20,23,24,28] Statistically significant reductions in triglyceride levels ranged from 0.3 to 0.89 mmol/L in participants with obesity, type 2 diabetes, or metabolic syndrome; however, one study reported no significant difference in triglyceride levels.[20,23,24,26] Most studies reported reduction in total cholesterol and LDL, but the impact on HDL cholesterol was mixed; in some interventions HDL cholesterol increased while in others it decreased.[23,24,27,28] One study reported unfavorable changes in total cholesterol and LDL cholesterol in a healthy population.[27]

GLYCEMIC CONTROL

Typically, fasting blood sugar and HbA1C are used to represent glycemic control. However, only one of the studies involving participants with type 2 diabetes or insulin resistance was long enough to measure change in HbA1C. In that 3-month intervention, the average HbA1C decreased from 6.6% to 6.2% in participants with type 2 diabetes.[20] Most studies did not report significant changes in fasting blood glucose.[23,26] A 2-week intervention in participants with type 2 diabetes improved insulin sensitivity by 1.3 M/LBM/l.[28]

OTHER OUTCOMES

Most studies that reported changes in systolic and/or diastolic blood pressure demonstrated modest reductions of 3–4 mm Hg; one study demonstrated reduction of 9.1 mm Hg in systolic blood pressure in a population with metabolic syndrome.[20,22–24] Significant changes in inflammation as measured by C-reactive protein (CRP) were not reported.[20,24] One study included an outcome of intestinal permeability with no significant change. When satiety was measured, the Paleolithic diets were shown to have increased satiety for energy density.[21,29]

PROS AND CONS

As with many popular diets, there are some redeeming factors on which the Paleo Diet is based, but there are some restrictive factors that are not fully supported by evidence. In terms of health benefits, the pros and cons include:

Pros

- The Paleo Diet emphasizes fruits and vegetables and is rich in most micronutrients; a diet rich in fruits and vegetables has many health benefits including risk reduction of cardiovascular disease and some forms of cancer.[30]
- The Paleo Diet encourages consumption of omega-3 fatty acids which have been suggested to have anti-inflammatory properties in the context of cardiovascular disease.[18]
- The Paleo Diet discourages consumption of processed foods and foods/beverages with added sugar; these foods and beverages can contribute to negative health outcomes.
- Several research studies have demonstrated that a Paleolithic diet improves glycemic control and cardiometabolic risk factors in people with type 2 diabetes, metabolic syndrome, and/or obesity.[19,20,22–24,28]

Cons

- The Paleo Diet discourages consumption of dairy products, whole grains, and legumes, which are food groups with nutritional benefits.

- The Paleo Diet can lead to inadequate intake of calcium and vitamin D.[7,22]
- Some studies have demonstrated a decrease in levels of HDL cholesterol following a Paleolithic diet intervention.[27,28]

Beyond the health benefits, it is important to consider the practicality of adhering to the Paleo Diet.

Pros

- The Paleo Diet does not require calorie counting, which eliminates an element of dieting that can be tedious for some people.
- The Paleo Diet requires very little weighing and measuring; only calorie-dense foods, such as dried fruit, nuts, and oils, are required to be measured.
- Depending upon the chosen level of adherence, there is some flexibility for choosing foods that are not part of the Paleo Diet.
- The popularity of the Paleo Diet has led to many cookbooks and recipes as well as recognition in the food industry, which can facilitate adherence to the diet.
- The Paleo Diet receives favorable scores for satiety, especially in terms of satiety for consumed energy.[21,29]

Cons

- The Paleo Diet restricts food groups that are commonly consumed, which can require extra planning when eating away from home.
- The Paleo Diet is not feasible for vegetarians or vegans.
- The amount of time required for meal preparation may be unrealistic for some people.
- One group of study participants rated the Paleo Diet more challenging to adhere to compared to the control diet.[21]
- The types of foods required by the Paleo Diet can be expensive; one study suggests that adherence to the Paleo Diet would increase a grocery bill by 10% over a comparable healthful diet.[31]

IS THIS DIET RIGHT FOR YOUR PATIENTS?

There is some evidence to suggest following the Paleo Diet can lead to short-term improvements in components of metabolic syndrome.[32] With proper guidance from a nutrition professional to ensure nutrient needs are being met, the Paleo Diet may be an effective diet intervention for people who have metabolic syndrome. However, any person considering the Paleo Diet should also take the following factors into consideration. To follow the Paleo Diet, a person must be willing to:

- Eat a diet heavy in meat
- Eat fruits and vegetables
- Avoid dairy, grains, and legumes
- Supplement vitamin D and possibly calcium
- Prepare meals at home and have access to space to store large amounts of meat and produce

Considering that improvements in metabolic markers occur in as few as 10–14 days, it would be possible to experiment with this diet pattern with short-term commitments. A more realistic, and likely more sustainable, approach would be to incorporate some of the principles of the Paleo Diet into a less strict diet. For example, increasing fruit and vegetable intake and decreasing intake of processed foods that contain added sugar and salt would be positive modifications to the traditional Western diet. It is not clear that whole grains, low-fat dairy, and legumes have to be eliminated from a diet for optimal control of metabolic factors.[32] Incorporating moderate amounts of these foods into a modified Paleolithic-style diet may be the most sustainable option. Ultimately, a diet to which a person can make a long-term commitment would have the greatest impact on lifelong health.

REFERENCES

1. Gans K. *Google's Most Popular Diets: 2014 Edition [Internet].* U.S. News & World Report. 2014 [cited 2016 Aug 11]. Available at: http://health.usnews.com/health-news/blogs/eat-run/2014/12/31/googles-most-popular-diets-2014-edition
2. Breslouer L. *Inside One of the Country's First Paleo Restaurants [Internet].* Thrillist. 2014 [cited 2016 Aug 11]. Available at: https://www.thrillist.com/eat/nation/paleo-restaurant-first-paleo-restaurant-in-america
3. Voegtlin WL. *The Stone Age Diet.* New York: Vantage Press; 1975.
4. Eaton SB, Konner M. Paleolithic nutrition. *N Engl J Med [Internet]* 1985;312(5):283–9. Available at: http://www.nejm.org/doi/abs/10.1056/NEJM198501313120505
5. Cordain L. [Internet] *The Paleo Diet.* 2016 [cited 2016 Aug 11]. Available at: http://thepaleodiet.com/dr-loren-cordain/
6. Cordain L. *The Paleo Diet.* New York: Wiley; 2002.
7. Cordain L. *The Paleo Diet: Lose Weight and Get Healthy by Eating the Foods You Were Designed to Eat.* Hoboken: John Wiley & Sons; 2010.
8. Revedin A, Aranguren B, Becattini R. et al. Thirty thousand-year-old evidence of plant food processing. *Proc Natl Acad Sci U S A* 2010;107(44):18815–9.
9. Mercader J. Mozambican grass seed consumption during the Middle Stone Age. *Science* 2009;326(5960):1680–3.
10. Sponheimer M, Alemseged Z, Cerling TE. et al. Isotopic evidence of early hominin diets. *Proc Natl Acad Sci [Internet]* 2013;110(26):10513–8. Available at: http://pubget.com/site/paper/23733964?institution=gwumc.edu%5Cnpapers3://publication/doi/10.1073/pnas.1222579110
11. Knight C. "Most people are simply not designed to eat pasta":1 evolutionary explanations for obesity in the low-carbohydrate diet movement. *Public Underst Sci [Internet]* 2011;20(5):706–19. Available at: http://journals.sagepub.com/doi/abs/10.1177/0963662511421711
12. Runyon J. The many types of paleo [Internet]. 2013. Available at: http://ultimatepaleoguide.com/many-types-of-paleo/
13. Miller J. The ultimate paleo guide to intermittent fasting [Internet]. 2015 [cited 2016 Aug 11]. Available at: http://ultimatepaleoguide.com/ultimate-paleo-guide-intermittent-fasting/
14. Gunnars K. A Paleo Diet Meal Plan and Menu That Can Save Your Life [Internet]. AuthorityNutrition.com. Available at: https://authoritynutrition.com/paleo-diet-meal-plan-and-menu/
15. Schwalfenberg GK. [Internet] The alkaline diet: Is there evidence that an alkaline pH diet benefits health? *J Environ Public Health* 2012; Article ID 727630.

16. Gearry RB, Irving PM, Barrett JS, Nathan DM, Shepherd SJ, Gibson PR. Reduction of dietary poorly absorbed short-chain carbohydrates (FODMAPs) improves abdominal symptoms in patients with inflammatory bowel disease—a pilot study. *J Crohn's Colitis [Internet]* 2009;3(1):8–14. Available at: http://dx.doi.org/10.1016/j.crohns.2008.09.004

17. Hou JK, Abrahama B, El-Serag H. Dietary intake and risk of developing inflammatory bowel disease: A systematic review of the literature. *Am J Gastroenterol* 2011;106:563–73.

18. Leaf A. Prevention of sudden cardiac death by n-3 polyunsaturated fatty acids. *J Cardiovasc Med* 2007;8(S1):S27–29.

19. Lindeberg S, Jönsson T, Granfeldt Y. et al. A Palaeolithic diet improves glucose tolerance more than a Mediterranean-like diet in individuals with ischaemic heart disease. *Diabetologia* 2007;50(9):1795–807.

20. Jonsson T, Granfeldt Y, Ahren B. et al. Beneficial effects of a Paleolithic diet on cardiovascular risk factors in type 2 diabetes: A randomized cross-over pilot study. *Cardiovasc Diabetol [Internet]* 2009;8(1):35. Available at: http://www.cardiab.com/content/8/1/35

21. Jönsson T, Granfeldt Y, Lindeberg S, Hallberg A-C. Subjective satiety and other experiences of a Paleolithic diet compared to a diabetes diet in patients with type 2 diabetes. *Nutr J [Internet]* 2013;12:105. Available at: http://www.pubmedcentral.nih.gov/articlerender.fcgi?artid=3727993&tool=pmcentrez&rendertype=abstract

22. Osterdahl M, Kocturk T, Koochek A, Wändell PE. Effects of a short-term intervention with a paleolithic diet in healthy volunteers. *Eur J Clin Nutr* 2008;62(5):682–5.

23. Frassetto LA, Schloetter M, Mietus-Synder M, Morris RC, Sebastian A. Metabolic and physiologic improvements from consuming a paleolithic, hunter-gatherer type diet. *Eur J Clin Nutr [Internet]* 2009;63(8):947–55. Available at: http://dx.doi.org/10.1038/ejcn.2009.4

24. Boers I, Muskiet FA, Berkelaar E. et al. Favourable effects of consuming a Palaeolithic-type diet on characteristics of the metabolic syndrome: A randomized controlled pilot-study. *Lipids Health Dis [Internet]* 2014;13:160. Available at: http://www.pubmedcentral.nih.gov/articlerender.fcgi?artid=4210559&tool=pmcentrez&rendertype=abstract

25. Whalen KA, McCullough M, Flanders WD, Hartman TJ, Judd S, Bostick RM. Paleolithic and Mediterranean diet pattern scores and risk of incident, sporadic colorectal adenomas. *Am J Epidemiol* 2014;180(11):1088–97.

26. Mellberg C, Sandberg S, Ryberg M. et al. Long-term effects of a Palaeolithic-type diet in obese postmenopausal women: A 2-year randomized trial. *Eur J Clin Nutr [Internet]* 2014;68(3):350–7. Available at: http://www.pubmedcentral.nih.gov/articlerender.fcgi?artid=4216932&tool=pmcentrez&rendertype=abstract

27. Smith M, Trexler E. Unrestricted Paleolithic diet is associated with unfavorable changes to blood lipids in healthy subjects. *Int J Exerc Sci [Internet]* 2014;7(46):128–39. Available at: http://digitalcommons.wku.edu/ijes/vol7/iss2/4/

28. Masharani U, Sherchan P, Schloetter M. et al. Metabolic and physiologic effects from consuming a hunter-gatherer (Paleolithic)-type diet in type 2 diabetes. *Eur J Clin Nutr [Internet]* 2015;69(November 2014):1–5. Available at: http://www.nature.com/doifinder/10.1038/ejcn.2015.39

29. Bligh HFJ, Godsland IF, Frost G. et al. Plant-rich mixed meals based on Palaeolithic diet principles have a dramatic impact on incretin, peptide YY and satiety response, but show little effect on glucose and insulin homeostasis: An acute-effects randomised study. *Br J Nutr [Internet]* 2015;113(4):574–84. Available at: http://www.ncbi.nlm.nih.gov/pubmed/25661189

30. Hung HC, Joshipura KJ, Jiang R. et al. Fruit and vegetable intake and risk of major chronic disease. *J Natl Cancer Inst* 2004;96(21):1577–84.

31. Metzgar M, Rideout TC, Fontes-Villalba M, Kuipers RS. The feasibility of a Paleolithic diet for low-income consumers. *Nutr Res [Internet]* 2011;31(6):444–51. Available at: http://dx.doi.org/10.1016/j.nutres.2011.05.008
32. Manheimer EW, Van Zuuren EJ, Fedorowicz Z, Pijl H. Paleolithic nutrition for metabolic syndrome: Systematic review and meta-analysis. *Am J Clin Nutr* 2015;102(4):922–32.

6 The South Beach Diet

Meghan Ariagno

CONTENTS

OVERVIEW

The South Beach Diet is a three-stage, modified low-carbohydrate diet plan designed to promote weight loss. It is introduced in the South Beach Diet book as a method for "Losing Weight, Gaining Life," and guarantees that with diet adherence, there is a decreased desire for unhealthy foods, which helps individuals control their cravings that can often sabotage weight loss efforts. Phase 1 is a two-week phase that eliminates most carbohydrates and emphasizes healthy, lean protein sources, high-fiber vegetables, and healthy fat sources. Phase 2 involves re-introducing some of the foods that were prohibited, such as whole-grain foods, fruits, and more vegetables. Phase 3 is a maintenance plan, meant to be followed for life.[1]

The South Beach Diet book became widely popular for consumers in 2003. It dominated the *New York Times* list of hardcover advice books and it was a bestseller book on Amazon.com.[2] Diet books offer consumers instant guidance and an action plan toward weight loss right at their fingertips, which likely drives their popularity. On the South Beach Diet, readers immediately are presented with promises of weight loss and are told, "you'll eat until your hunger is satisfied," while being on a diet that "saves your life," by helping your cardiovascular system.[1] At the time this book was published, consumers had both positive and negative associations with carbohydrates due to mixed messages from the advertising industry and medical community. Some negative qualities included, "carbohydrates make you fat, raise insulin levels, and slow down your metabolism."[3] Hence, many people were willing to follow a low-carbohydrate diet in hopes of weight loss.

The creator of the diet, Dr. Arthur Agatston, describes the South Beach Diet as a diet that promotes eating the right carbohydrates and the right fats. He does not claim the diet to be either low-carbohydrate or low fat in design. This formula, he believes, is meant to support long-term weight loss that is sustainable. By emphasizing foods that slow the process of digestion (high-fiber carbohydrates, protein, and healthy fats), control of appetite is better achieved. Eating "bad" carbohydrates (or highly processed carbohydrates) creates cravings for more "bad" carbohydrates. He believes this is primarily responsible for the obesity epidemic. Dr. Agatston believes that most of the excess weight people accumulate is due to overconsumption of processed carbohydrates such as baked goods, breads, and refined foods. White flour and white sugar are banned from the South Beach Diet, but whole grain breads, cereals, and whole-wheat pasta are allowed. The South Beach Diet proudly stands apart from low-fat, heart-healthy diets by allowing lean beef, pork, veal, and lamb. The healthier fats, from mono- and polyunsaturated sources, are encouraged, not only for their health benefits, but also for their palatability and satiation effects. These include items like avocado, olive oil, and nuts.[1]

Dr. Agatston, a Cardiologist, noticed his patients did not see the cholesterol-lowering effect from the American Heart Association's recommendations to follow a low-fat diet. He quickly tried to separate the South Beach Diet message from other popular diet messages of the time. The Atkins Diet is considered a high-protein diet and the Ornish Diet emphasizes a low-fat diet but does not include healthy fat sources. Low carbohydrate diet trends started with the introduction of the Atkins Diet and the Zone Diet in the mid-1990s. Reducing carbohydrates has sound reasoning for weight management as well as heart health. Although controversial, highly refined, processed carbohydrates may play a larger role than saturated fats in promoting poor cardiovascular health.[4]

The South Beach Diet Super Charged, was published in 2008. It is an updated version of the original South Beach Diet that not only emphasizes a three phase diet plan, but also outlines a three phase workout strategy with the collaboration of Dr. Joseph Signorile, a professor of exercise physiology at the University of Miami. Exercise is not emphasized greatly in the original South Beach Diet book, but it is included in the updated version. Readers are instructed to participate in 20 minutes of daily exercise that alternates between walking and a strength-training workout to help boost metabolism and prevent weight plateaus. There is also optional support available online at a cost. There is access to a weight-loss tracker, printable shopping list, daily newsletter, and an online community message board.[5] Currently, the South Beach Diet website (www.southbeachdiet.com) offers the ability to follow the program while having prepared food delivered while being a part of an online community.

HOW THE DIET WORKS

The South Beach Diet consists of three phrases. The instructions state to eat "three balanced meals" and to eat until hunger is satisfied by following the outlined meal plans and using the recipes provided. Consuming three snacks throughout the day is also encouraged (mid-morning, mid-afternoon, and after dinner). There are no calorie counts one has to follow. Carbohydrate amount is varied throughout all three phases. The diet emphasizes protein and healthy fats and as the diet progresses, the presence of high-fiber carbohydrate gradually increases.[1] See Table 6.1 for a brief outline.[6]

TABLE 6.1
Overview of the South Beach Diet

Duration of Treatment	Energy Intake	% Protein	% Carbohydrate	% Fat	Low Carb	Low Fat	Alcohol Intake	Caffeine Intake
Phase 1: 2 weeks	Not specified	25–30	20–30 Carbohydrate amount gradually increases through each stage	40–50	Yes	No	Wine is allowed	No restriction
Phase 2: Until target weight is achieved								
Phase 3: Lifelong maintenance								

Source: Atallah R. et al. *Circ Cardiovasc Qual Outcomes* 2014;7:815–842.

PHASE ONE

This is the strictest phase of the diet, lasting for two weeks. It emphasizes protein and healthy fat sources. The purpose of this phase is to help regulate blood sugar and insulin resistance. By doing so, as explained in the book, unhealthy cravings will decrease.[1]

Despite the rigidity of these first two weeks, the diet promises the body will adjust to the strict avoidance of certain carbohydrates. The diet starts with as little as 20 g of carbohydrate daily on Phase One and gradually increases during each stage.[7] There are meal plans outlined for all 14 days while on Phase One, along with recipes as well as food lists for "foods to enjoy" and "foods to avoid."

Foods permitted on this stage include meat, chicken, turkey, fish, shellfish, eggs, cheese, vegetables, and nuts. Olive oil is promoted to accompany salads. Foods that are excluded on this stage include bread, rice, potatoes, and pasta. Also, fruit and dairy are to be avoided due to their carbohydrate amount. Desserts, such as candy, cake, cookies, ice cream, baked goods, sugar, and alcohol, are all excluded.[1]

PHASE TWO

Advancing to this stage liberalizes the amounts of carbohydrates and sweets allowed but in a controlled way. The duration of this stage is meant to be as long as is needed to reach the desired goal weight. It is recommended to gradually reintroduce carbohydrates to avoid big swings in blood sugar. Fibrous foods (fruits, whole grains, etc.) are recommended. Readers are also alerted to limit intake of high glycemic index foods while on this stage. Examples include: carrots, banana, watermelon, and pineapple. Similar to Phase One, this stage has 14 meal plans, with accompanying recipes and lists for "foods to enjoy" and "foods to avoid." Readers go into this stage understanding that their weight loss will slow down.

It is suggested in Phase Two that every individual will experience this phase differently. For example, bread may be a trigger food that could lead to increased cravings for some people, while pasta may do the same for others. Different carbo-hydrates may cause different effects in hunger and cravings and it is up to the individual to understand this and make adjustments to their intake as needed. Readers are also given a relapse tip: In case there is a slip in dieting efforts (examples include overindulging on a vacation or during the holidays), going back to Phase One is allowed just until the weight that was gained is lost.[1]

Keys to success[1]

- Try every recipe
- Avoid having fruit with breakfast
- Take advantage of all the foods and ingredients
- Use all herbs and spices
- Be open to creative substitutions for cravings
- Eat something 15 minutes before arriving at a restaurant
- Order soup as a first course at a restaurant (clear broth or consommé)

PHASE THREE

This phase is meant to be a lifetime plan and reaching this point means an individual has reached their ideal weight. This is the most liberal stage of the diet. At this phase, an individual can consume about 30% of their calories from carbohydrates daily. This stage does not have a "foods to avoid" list because indulging is permitted, but in a controlled way. Included in this phase are 14 meal plans and recipes. As stated earlier, a person can go back to Phase One if weight gain occurs while in Phase Three. The diet stands by the principles of flexibility and simplicity. There are tips discussed throughout the book. For example, while on Phase Three, dieters are encouraged to avoid skipping breakfast. Also, calorie counting, weighing food, and measuring portion sizes is not a focus of the South Beach Diet. The one exception is participants are instructed to always portion out nuts, oils, hummus, and other fat sources. (Example: 15 almonds or cashews or 30 pistachios).[1]

EXERCISE

The South Beach Diet promises to be effective despite the activity or exercise habits of individuals. While the South Beach Diet lacks the structured exercise plan outlined in *The South Beach Diet Super Charged,* it does promote a sound message regarding exercise. Exercise should not feel like it is interfering with one's whole life. Instead, establishing a routine that can be incorporated in one's lifestyle is recommended. While one may not achieve the greatest caloric burn with a lower intensity exercise plan as compared to a higher intensity workout, if it is something that can be maintained consistently, the benefits carry a greater effect. Agatston recommends a workout as minimal as a 20-minute brisk walk every day. He also encourages maintaining a regular stretching routine. Last, he encourages participating in weight training. He does not define specific frequency goals, but ties in the benefits of strength training to help support metabolism and maintain bone density.[1]

CURRENT RESEARCH

Diet books often include non-evidence-based information and health promises that can be misleading to the consumer. To help understand the South Beach Diet's claims more rigorously, research was gathered on other themes presented in the book (high-protein diets, glycemic index, and appetite control). Research is limited on the South Beach Diet. While the diet does suggest it is helpful with short-term weight loss, there is little evidence on the long-term effects of the diet on weight loss and weight maintenance.

The diet claims that most people lose 8–13 pounds within the first two weeks, followed by a 1–2 pound loss per week. Goff and colleagues evaluated a variety of the nutrition statements presented in the South Beach Diet book and using peer-reviewed literature, determined the validity of the statements. The promises of the proven effectiveness of the diet and that the "first 2 weeks yields a weight loss of 8–13 pounds," could not be supported by peer-reviewed literature. Forty-two nutrition facts were included in their evaluation. Fourteen (33%) facts were supported, 7 (17%) were not supported, 18 (43%) were both supported and not supported, and 3 (7%) had no related papers, including the fact that the diet had been "scientifically studied and proven effective."[2]

The South Beach Diet does emphasize protein sources throughout all three phases.

Per evidence-based medicine, high-protein diets (1.2–1.6 g/kg) have been associated with weight loss success.[8] Dietary protein has a higher thermic effect than carbohydrates and fat. Protein requires about 20%–30% of available energy for its metabolism and storage, whereas carbohydrates require 5%–10% and dietary fats require 3% or less. While weight loss leads to a decrease in resting metabolic rate, higher-protein diets may slow the reduction in the resting metabolic rate. Additionally, protein's role in achieving greater satiety feelings are well documented.[7,9,10]

The South Beach Diet recommends choosing carbohydrates that are low on the glycemic index. Currently, there is no standard definition of a low-glycemic index or low-glycemic load diet. The glycemic index classifies the quality of carbohydrates and includes a rating system based on the rise in blood glucose levels two hours after consumption. A low-glycemic index diet has not been associated with increased weight loss.[7] The European Food Safety Authority claims there is insufficient scientific evidence to support low-glycemic index diets as a weight management strategy. A meta-analysis conducted on 6 randomized controlled trials (RCTs) including 202 subjects who were randomly assigned to dietary interventions with durations varying between five weeks or six months showed that a low-glycemic index diet had a greater effect on weight loss than a high-glycemic index diet. However, the studies did not adjust for potential confounders such as protein or total fiber so this data has limitations for interpretation.[11] Last, in the recent position paper from the Academy of Nutrition and Dietetics for Interventions for the Treatment of Overweight and Obesity in Adults, the data was poor to support a low-glycemic index diet for weight management without also providing caloric restriction.[12]

Beyond calorie reduction, hormones and peptides play a role in body weight regulation. Appetite is regulated by innumerable variables, including the following hormones: leptin, ghrelin, cholecystokinin, peptide YY, insulin, pancreatic polypeptide, and glucagon-like peptide 1 (GLP-1). Leptin's role is to signal the hypothalamus to reduce food intake. Ghrelin stimulates hunger while Peptide YY, GLP-1, cholecystokinin, pancreatic polypeptide, and amylin inhibit intake and promote satiety. These peptides are stimulated by dietary protein, among other dietary components.[8] When calories are restricted, there is an acute compensatory pattern of these hormones that favors weight regain. For example, when energy expenditure, levels of leptin, and cholecystokinin are reduced, there is an increase in ghrelin and subsequently, appetite.[13] Reducing calories will likely promote weight loss for most. However, the majority of dieters will unfortunately fail to maintain the weight that has been lost due to these alterations in appetite and fullness signals. Changes can persist for 12 months after weight loss, Sumithran and colleagues noted.[13] That being said, it is helpful to provide support for any individual who has been successful with weight loss (following any diet) to help minimize weight regain. Therefore, a weight loss of 1–2 lbs per week as promised by the South Beach Diet may not be attainable by all, especially after 12 months of following the diet plan.

Research has suggested that low-carbohydrate diets promote greater weight loss than low-fat diets in the short term (six months). However, after 12 months, the weight loss difference between the two diet regimens is not maintained.[7,14] Long-term randomized controlled trials show similar weight loss results for both low-carbohydrate and low-fat diets.[9] As carbohydrates are broken down, glucose enters the bloodstream and insulin is released. Insulin will promote fatty acid synthesis and storage. When following a reduced carbohydrate diet, the metabolic effect may favor a reduction in fatty acid synthesis and fat storage.[9] Although there may be a short-term benefit to reducing carbohydrates for weight loss, research does not prove its effectiveness in the long term.

TYPICAL RESULTS

There is limited research evaluating the weight loss results with the South Beach Diet. As stated earlier, the book claims that during the first two weeks in Phase One, expected weight loss is between 8 and 13 pounds. This claim has not been supported. In Phase Two, people may lose, on average, one to two pounds per week. In 2014, Atallah and colleagues compared the effectiveness of the Atkins, South Beach, Weight Watchers, and Zone Diets. Focus was centered on the sustainability of weight loss at ≥ 1 year. Each diet yielded comparable weight loss results of about 5% total body weight loss from baseline weight by 12 months, with some weight regain occurring by two years.[6]

The evidence for a specific distribution of macronutrients to support weight loss has also not been elucidated. Various amounts of macronutrient composition were examined in the POUNDS (Prevention of Obesity Using Novel Dietary Strategies (POUNDS) LOST Study using four different diets. Weight loss occurred in all groups. Within 1 year of initiating the diet, weight loss plateaued. After two years, some, but not all, experienced some form of weight regain. This study illustrated an important finding that general adherence to a calorie-controlled diet was the major determinant of weight loss, rather than adherence to a specific macronutrient composition.[15]

The question of why people may fail on the South Beach Diet is discussed in the book. With any diet over the long-term, individuals get tired of the rigidity of following a diet and deviate on their own. Lifestyle factors may pose a challenge as well, such as traveling frequently for work or needing to prepare food for other family members who are not following the diet plan. In these cases, adherence may be difficult.[1]

Factors that contribute to successful maintenance of weight loss have included the following: adherence to a low-fat diet, frequent self-monitoring of body weight (daily or weekly) and food intake, high levels of physical activity, and long-term patient-provider contact.[7] The South Beach Diet does not endorse all of these features so while there may be elements of the diet that are useful and appealing, promoting more self-monitoring and/or emphasizing higher levels of activity may enhance an individual's success.

PROS

Short-lasting Phase One

- Consistent dietary and lifestyle changes are more likely to be successful when the diet plan is balanced and moderate.[16] That being said, once dieters reach Phase Two (after two weeks on Phase One), the diet begins to resemble a more "normal" style of eating.
- The balanced plan consists of protein, fiber, and healthy fats. There is also an emphasis on including unprocessed wholesome foods, such as including steel cut oatmeal instead of instant oatmeal. Protein's benefits have been mentioned earlier.

Emphasis on dietary fiber

- Populations that include more fiber in their daily diets have lower body weights. The average American does not meet the daily-recommended consumption of fiber of approximately 25–38 grams/daily.[17] However, in the literature, in regards to body mass index (BMI), both normal BMI and overweight BMI individuals consume more fiber on average compared to individuals with obesity. Research from the International Study of Macro-/Micronutrients and Blood Pressure (INTERMAP) make a connection between low intakes of dietary fiber and higher body mass index. Also, the Nurses' Health Study and Nurses' Health Study II data demonstrate the protective benefits of whole grain consumption and avoiding weight gain.[17] Beginning with Phase Two, fiber sources have a greater presence in the diet, and with that come additional health benefits. Markers of cardiovascular disease (triglycerides and high-density lipoprotein cholesterol) are improved with low-carbohydrate diets as compared with low-fat diets.[9]

Emphasis on healthy fats

- Emphasizing healthy fat in the diet is important because it aids in the absorption of fat-soluble nutrients and provides essential fatty acids.[18]

Recipes

- The South Beach Diet book provides many recipes to follow, all with simple ingredients. There are multiple cookbooks to purchase or recipe collections that are also available online.[25]

Restaurant Eating Tips

- There are useful tips for managing eating out at restaurants. Dieting can often lead individuals to feel they cannot be social or that all meals at restaurants will sabotage their weight loss efforts. While certainly some menus may be limited in their healthy food offerings, there are no shortages of strategies that can be helpful in supporting weight control.
  1. Eat a small snack before arriving at a restaurant
  2. Avoid the bread
  3. Fill up on a soup
  4. Order a double serving of vegetables
- These tips provide individuals the confidence in knowing that even when they may not be in control of food preparation, they can still enjoy a social occasion and a healthier restaurant eating experience.[1]

CONS

Limited emphasis on lifestyle approach

- While the South Beach Diet promises that pounds will be lost, achieving success with weight management needs to go beyond the scale. Emphasis needs to be placed on the development of healthful lifestyles that can be sustained over the long term with a focus on overall fitness and health.[19]

Limited encouragement of interaction with health-focused health professional

- With many popular diets that are self-initiated and implemented, there is no coaching or counseling from a health professional to provide support and guidance. Research continues to support the importance of provider/client contact toward a successful diet intervention.[8] The 2013 American Heart Association/American College of Cardiology/and The Obesity Society (AHA/ACC/TOS) guidelines for the management of overweight and obesity in adults suggests that the most effective behavioral weight loss treatment is an in-person, high-intensity (i.e., ≥14 sessions in six months) comprehensive weight loss intervention provided in individual or group sessions by a trained interventionist.[20]
- During the sessions, discussions can be initiated for behavioral modification interventions for weight loss. These may include goal setting, promoting self-monitoring, cognitive restructuring, and strategies centered around stimulus control and relapse prevention.[7]
- Another advantage in working with a health professional is to establish a healthy goal weight and a safe number of pounds of weight to lose per week. Individuals may expect to achieve a certain low body weight while following the South Beach Diet that may be unrealistic. Despite achieving some weight loss, individuals may feel like a failure if it does not align with a predetermined goal.

Lack of an "individual approach"

- Jortberg and colleagues emphasized the key to successful weight management is an individualized approach, which the South Beach Diet does not emphasize. There is no interpretation of an individual's food preferences, cultural considerations, or environmental and schedule challenges.[19]
- If individuals are placed on a structured diet that may not align with their typical food patterns or selection, they may be missing the specific cause(s) of their weight gain and thus be unable to address the changes required to be successful. If the diet is abandoned, and no efforts are made to modify original eating behaviors, an individual's risk of weight regain may be high.[21]

IS THIS DIET RIGHT FOR YOUR PATIENTS?

Due to the rising obesity rates, many individuals are taking it on themselves to look for programs and/or support for weight loss. They no longer need to seek dietary advice from qualified health professionals and the plentiful amount of information available may not be science-based.[22] Individuals may perceive their best chance for weight loss is to restrict their carbohydrate intake. Many people perceive low-carbohydrate diets to be a healthy way to lose weight.[23] For some individuals, completely restricting certain foods is easier than achieving a form of moderation so taking an approach similar to the South Beach Diet seems manageable.[3]

The Academy of Nutrition and Dietetics, the world's largest organization of food and nutrition professionals, promotes evidence-based recommendations for weight loss. There are elements of the South Beach Diet that may work for some individuals. The menus available in the book make it very manageable to follow and the diet is even more manageable if one chooses to have their meals delivered following the online program. However, this is also an added expense. To enhance success, individuals may benefit from the added support by meeting regularly with an RDN to discuss individual goals and establish an exercise plan. While the rigidity of Phase One may not be appealing to all, having the support of nutrition counseling may help an individual's success. Phase Two and beyond is a more balanced and realistic approach to weight loss and may help support people toward their weight and health goals. The diet becomes much more flexible and realistic, and as a result may be more attractive for individuals.

Depending on whether someone chooses to follow the South Beach Diet on their own or using their online, prepared food delivery service, the diet does offer advantages for people who choose to avoid refined foods. Other important points to consider would be one's financial situation and how accessible fresh fruits, vegetables, lean protein sources, and whole grains are. Although there is not the expense of supplements, the emphasis of produce may be a higher expense for some individuals. Food deserts, or "grocery gaps," are areas without adequate supermarkets or farmers' markets offering healthy and affordable foods. Similar to other commercialized weight-loss programs, the offering of healthy food with no preparation needed could be a great value for busy, on-the-go families or professionals.

The best weight management approach involves adoption and maintenance of life-style behaviors contributing to both dietary intake and physical activity.[12] Pursuing weight loss with unrealistic goals in mind may interfere with achieving any weight loss success.[24] A realistic goal for weight loss is a 5%–10% reduction within six months.[12]

An individual's success with the South Beach Diet may be enhanced by including nutrition counseling with a Registered Dietitian Nutritionist (RDN). These counseling sessions could provide an opportunity to discuss goal setting and behavior change in a more tailored and individualized way. For example, through motivational interviewing, individuals can feel supported through their diet and lifestyle changes. These sessions could allow for opportunities to increase nutrition knowledge as well as review coping strategies or create a plan that incorporates preferential foods in a healthful and appropriate manner.[16]

REFERENCES

1. Agatston A. *The South Beach Diet: The Delicious, Doctor-Designed, Foolproof Plan for Fast and Healthy Weight Loss.* New York: Random House; 2003.
2. Goff SL, Foody JM, Inzucchi S. et al. Brief report: Nutrition and weight loss information in a popular diet book: Is it fact, fiction, or something in between? *J Gen Intern Med* 2006;21:769–774.
3. Levine M, Jones J, Lineback D. Low-carbohydrate diets: Assessing the science and knowledge gaps, summary of an ILSI North America workshop. *J Am Diet Assoc* 2006;106(12):2086–2094.
4. Stein K. Severely restricted diets in the absence of medical necessity: The unintended consequences. *J Acad Nutr Diet* 2014;114(7):986–994.
5. South Beach Diet Supercharged. South Beach Diet Online. http://www.southbeachdiet.com/diet/south-beach-diet-supercharged-book. Accessed August, 2016.
6. Atallah R, Filion K, Wakil S. et al. Long-term effects of 4 popular diets on weight loss and cardiovascular risk factors. A systematic review of randomized controlled trials. *Circ Cardiovasc Qual Outcomes* 2014;7:815–842.
7. Eckel R. Nonsurgical management of obesity in adults. *N Engl J Med* 2008;358:1941–1950.
8. Leidy HJ, Clifton PM, Astrup A. et al. The role of protein in weight loss and maintenance. *Am J Clin Nutr* 2015;101:1320S–1329S.
9. Hite AH, Berkowitz G, Berkowitz K. Low-carbohydrate diet review: Shifting the paradigm. *J Parenter Neteral Nutr* 2011;26(3):300–308.
10. Dhillon J, Craig BA, Leidy H. et al. The effects of increased protein intake on fullness: A meta-analysis and its limitations. *J Acad Nutr Diet* 2016;116(6):968–983.
11. Juanola-Falgarona M, Salas-Salvadó J, Ibarrola-Jurado N. et al. Effect of the glycemic index of the diet on weight loss, modulation of satiety, inflammation, and other metabolic risk factors: A randomized controlled trial. *Am J Clin Nutr* 2014;100(1):27–35.
12. Raynor H, Champagne C. Position of the academy of nutrition and dietetics: Interventions for the treatment of overweight and obesity in adults. *J Acad Nutr Diet* 2016;116(1):129–147.
13. Sumithran P, Prendergast L, Delbridge E. et al. Long-term persistence of hormonal adaptations to weight loss. *N Engl J Med* 2011;365:1597–1604.
14. Malik VS, Hu F. Popular weight-loss diets: From evidence to practice. *Nat Clin Pract* 2007;4(1):34–41.
15. Champagne C, Kris-Etherton P, Raynor H, Wolf A. What and when to eat…what works for obesity treatment? *Weight Management Matters; Winter* 2015;13(1):8–11.

16. Freeland-Graves J, Nitzke S. Position of the academy of nutrition and dietetics: Total approach to healthy eating. *J Acad Nutr Diet* 2013;113:307–317.
17. Dahl WJ, Stewart ML. Position of the academy of nutrition and dietetics: Health implications of dietary fiber. *J Acad Nutr Diet* 2015;115(11):1861–1870.
18. Vannice G, Rasmusseen H. Position of the academy of nutrition and dietetics: Dietary fatty acids for healthy adults. *J Acad Nutr Diet* 2014;114(1):136–153.
19. Jortberg B, Myers E, Gigliotti L. et al. Academy of nutrition and dietetics: Standards of practice and standards of professional performance for registered dietitian nutritionists (Competent, proficient, and expert) in adult weight management. *J Acad Nutr Diet* 2015;115(4):609–618.
20. Jensen M, Ryan D, Apovian C. et al. 2013 AHA/ACC/TOS guideline for the management of overweight and obesity in adults. A report of the American College of Cardiology/American Heart Association. *J AM Coll Cardiol* 2014;63(25):2985–3023.
21. Mozaffarian D, Hao T, Rimm E. et al. Changes in diet and lifestyle and long-term weight gain in women and men. *N Engl J Med* 2011;364:2393–2404.
22. Ayoob KT, Duyff R, Quagliani D. et al. Position of the American Dietetic Association: Food and nutrition misinformation. *J Am Diet Assoc* 2002;102(2):260–266.
23. Finny Rutten LJ, Yaroch AL, Colón-Ramos U. et al. Awareness, use and perceptions of low-carbohydrate diets. *Prev Chronic Dis* 2008;5(4):A130.
24. Cunningham E. How can I support my clients in setting realistic weight loss goals? *J Acad Nutr Diet* 2014;114:176.
25. The South Beach Diet Online https://www.southbeachdiet.com/home/index.jsp Accessed August 15, 2016.

7 Vegan Diets

Sai Krupa Das, Micaela C. Karlsen,
Caroline Blanchard, and Susan B. Roberts

CONTENTS

OVERVIEW

The hallmark of vegan diets is the absence of animal products including meat, poultry, milk, and fish. Relatively few Americans follow a vegan diet, with just 2% currently self-reporting as vegan adherents,[1] up from 1% in the 1970s.[2] However, the growing body of research reporting health and environmental benefits of vegan dietary patterns is likely to increase the number of individuals interested in adhering to a vegan dietary pattern. In particular, adherence to a vegan diet is associated with weight loss in overweight adults.[3,4] In addition, there are clear benefits of vegan eating for reduced greenhouse gas emissions and water use for food production.[5] For example, beef production uses 20 times more water than grain and root vegetable agriculture per calorie of food produced,[6] and systems modeling indicates that worldwide use of plant-based diets that align with current nutrition guidelines could reduce greenhouse gas emissions due to food by 29%–70%.[7]

There are three broadly different subtypes of vegan diets: vegan (general), raw food vegan, and whole food vegan, which differ from other common dietary patterns that exclude meat as summarized in Table 7.1. Most research on health benefits has been conducted using the whole food, plant-based vegan diet, which generally has the best micronutrient profile of the different vegan diets and is also low in fat due to the restriction of added oils. Multiple studies indicate that the use of this dietary pattern is associated with moderate weight loss without the need for portion control,[3,4,8] and some studies also indicate significant improvements in cardiometabolic risk factors and glycemic control. In addition, evidence from one research group suggests the potential for the combination of vegan diets, exercise, and meditation to reverse atherosclerosis.[9]

TABLE 7.1

Included and Excluded Food Groups in Self-Identified Vegetarian Dietary Patterns

Self-Identified Dietary Pattern	Pattern Excludes	Pattern Emphasizes
Vegetarian	All meat, including red meat, poultry, and usually fish	Whole grains, fruits, vegetables, legumes, nuts, and seeds. Does not "emphasize," but many vegetarians do eat processed foods. Some people may or may not eat fish, eggs, cheese.
Pescatarian	Red meat and poultry	Fish, whole grains, fruits, vegetables, legumes, nuts and seeds. Does not "emphasize," but many vegetarians do eat processed foods. Some people may or may not eat eggs and cheese.
Vegan (general)	All meat (red, poultry, fish) & dairy	Raw and cooked whole grains, fruits, vegetables, legumes, nuts, and seeds. May include processed foods, refined oils, and carbohydrates.
Raw Vegan	All meat, fish and dairy, cooked food, and usually processed food	Raw vegetables, fruits, nuts and seeds, soaked grains, and nuts. This is often a higher-fat diet because of larger quantities of nuts.
Whole Food Vegan	All meat (red, poultry, fish), dairy, processed food, added sugar, added oil, added/high salt	Raw and cooked whole grains, fruits, vegetables, legumes, nuts, and seeds. This is usually a low-fat diet because of the absence of refined oils.

These beneficial effects of low-fat vegan dietary patterns are complex and unlikely to be due to any single dietary factor.[10] It also is important to note the potential negative effects of a vegan diet, including increased risk of deficiencies of several nutrients such as vitamin B12, vitamin E, calcium, zinc, iron, and the essential fatty acids docosahexaenoic acid (DHA) and eicosapentaenoic acid (EPA).[11–13]

HOW TO FOLLOW A VEGAN DIET

Individuals considering adopting a vegan diet need to first decide the type of vegan diet they will follow. There are numerous books and websites that have suggested meal plans and recipes for each type of eating program. In addition, online support groups provide peer advice to help new members make the transition from a with-meat to a without-meat eating plan, and also suggest smartphone applications that help identify vegan-friendly restaurants. It can be challenging to make the changes required to adopt a vegan eating pattern both at home and when eating out. The challenges of eating out are particularly significant, as most restaurants do not cater to vegans. Nevertheless, label reading, calling ahead to request a special dish, and ordering vegetarian options with the additional request to remove items such as eggs and cheese are practical strategies that can work in any restaurant. Many traditional cuisines that emphasize vegetables with rice, such as Chinese, Japanese, Thai, Vietnamese, and Korean, are relatively easy to customize to fit a vegan diet. Alternatively, American-style restaurants and steakhouses often have baked potatoes, salad bars, and vegetable sides that can be assembled for a complete meal. A 2009 study suggested that being randomized to consume a vegan dietary pattern was no more difficult than following another medically recommended diet,[14] but the population was comprised by individuals who were ready to enroll in a challenging research study and may have underestimated the commitment needed by individuals who do not have some separately motivating factors for vegan eating, such as religion, a passion for animal welfare, or global warming. However, it is likely that as the demand for vegan foods increases, there will be a market response to cater to this need, similar to the recent demand for gluten-free products.

TYPICAL MENU PLANS

The following examples illustrate typical menus and calculated nutrient profiles for individuals following vegan (general), raw food vegan, and whole food vegan diets. In addition, an example of a vegan menu including processed foods of low nutritional quality is provided to illustrate the fact that diets devoid of animal products may not necessarily be inherently healthy; instead, their health quotient depends on the specific plant-based foods that are selected.

Also as noted below, although day-to-day variation in eating patterns will allow for fluctuations in micronutrient intakes, all vegans should supplement their diet with vitamin B12 and some with vitamin D in consultation with the individual's primary care physician.

Example vegan (general) menu			
Breakfast	Oatmeal with vanilla sweetened soymilk, ground flaxseed, walnuts, maple syrup, and orange juice		
Snack	Apple and peanut butter		
Lunch	Chipotle tofu sofritas burrito		
Snack	Carrot cake bar		
Dinner	Tofu-vegetable stir fry with brown rice		
Energy (kcal)	1819		
% kcal from protein	13		
% kcal from carbohydrate	56		
% kcal from fat	31		
% kcal from saturated fat	6		
Fiber (g)	36		
Italicized values are less than the recommended amounts for women 31–50[15]	Micronutrient	Content	Unit
	Vitamin A (total retinol activity equivalents)	*626*	*μg*
	Vitamin D	*2.3*	*μg*
	Vitamin E (total alpha-tocopherol equivalents)	22	mg
	Vitamin K	133	μg
	Vitamin C	208	mg
	Thiamin	1.5	mg
	Riboflavin	1.7	mg
	Niacin (equivalents)	32	mg

	Vitamin B6	2.4	mg
	Folate (equivalents)	432	mcg
	Vitamin B12	*1.9*	*µg*
	Calcium	1127	mg
	Phosphorus	1275	mg
	Magnesium	528	mg
	Iron	19	mg
	Zinc	10	mg
	Sodium	2783	mg
	Potassium	*3498*	*mg*
	Supplements needed to ensure adequacy relative to recommendations for woman aged 30–55 years: vitamin B12 and vitamin D.		

Comment on vegan (general) menu example: Vitamin A and potassium were low in this example but are not generally low in this menu plan—there is variability across different foods and while this single day example is low, anticipated values would be above recommended amounts on average, such that only vitamin B12 and vitamin D need to be routinely supplemented.

Example Raw Food Vegan menu			
Breakfast	Blueberry-kale smoothie (blueberry, kale, banana, orange, water, ground flaxseed)		
Snack	Raw oats, almonds, raisins		
Lunch	Large salad of mixed greens, kale, carrots, broccoli, zucchini, apple, beets, walnut pate (walnuts, tamari, parsley, dates, mustard)		
Snack	3 bananas		
Dinner	Large salad of sweet corn,[2] sugar snap peas, jicama, parsley, sunflower seeds, sweet red pepper, flax oil, vinegar		
Energy (kcal)	1833		
% kcal from protein	7		
% kcal from carbohydrate	60		
% kcal from fat	32		
% kcal from saturated fat	3		
Fiber (g)	60		
Italicized values are less than the recommended amounts for women 31–50[15]	Micronutrient	Content	Unit
	Vitamin A (total retinol activity equivalents)	1931	mcg
	Vitamin D	*0*	*mcg*
	Vitamin E (total alpha-tocopherol equivalents)	19	mg

Vitamin K	2404	mcg
Vitamin C	617	mg
Thiamin	1.5	mg
Riboflavin	1.6	mg
Niacin (equivalents)	24	mg
Vitamin B6	3.8	mg
Folate (equivalents)	820	mcg
Vitamin B12	*0*	*mcg*
Calcium	*629*	*mg*
Phosphorus	998	mg
Magnesium	570	mg
Iron	18	mg
Zinc	8	mg
Sodium	606	mg
Potassium	5433	mg
Supplements needed to ensure adequacy relative to recommendations for woman aged 30–55 years: vitamin B12, vitamin D, and calcium.		

Comment on raw food vegan menu example: This example is low in calcium as well as vitamin B12 and vitamin D, which may be typical due to the higher proportion of calories derived from fat.

Example Whole Food Vegan menu	
Breakfast	Steel cut oatmeal with fortified, unsweetened almond milk, apple, raisins, ground flaxseed
Snack	Carrot sticks and hummus
Lunch	Large salad of spinach, mixed greens, cooked kale, tomato, cucumber, quinoa, sweet potato, black beans, walnuts, lemon-tahini dressing
Snack	Chia pudding with berries and lime
Dinner	Kale and white-bean soup with brown rice
Energy (kal)	1858
% kcal from protein	14
% kcal from carbohydrate	69
% kcal from fat	17
% kcal from saturated fat	2
Fiber (g)	74

Italicized values are less than the recommended amounts for women 31–50[15]	Micronutrient	Content	Unit
	Vitamin A (total retinol activity equivalents)	3150	mcg
	Vitamin D	*1.3*	*mcg*
	Vitamin E (total alpha-tocopherol equivalents)	14	mg
	Vitamin K	1827	mcg
	Vitamin C	196	mg
	Thiamin	10	mg
	Riboflavin	9	mg
	Niacin (equivalents)	65	mg
	Vitamin B6	82	mg
	Folate (equivalents)	900	mcg
	Vitamin B12	6.6	mcg
	Calcium	*845*	*mg*
	Phosphorus	1869	mg
	Magnesium	745	mg
	Iron	24	mg
	Zinc	16	mg
	Sodium	800	mg
	Potassium	4663	mg
	Supplements needed to ensure adequacy relative to recommendations for woman aged 30–55 years: vitamin B12 and vitamin D.		

Comment on whole food vegan menu example: In general, fewer micronutrients are deficient in this eating plan compared with other vegan menus. For example, in this menu, vitamin B12 is not below recommended intake values; however, as a matter of principle, all vegans are recommended to take vitamin B12, so the vitamin, along with vitamin D, is included as a recommended supplement.

Example vegan menu including processed foods of low nutritional quality	
Breakfast	Sweetened corn and oat cereal with sweetened fortified soymilk
Snack	White chocolate & nut bar
Lunch	Veggie burger (fast food), French fries with ketchup, and soda
Snack	Potato chips and cookies
Dinner	White pasta with marinara sauce
Energy	1879
% kcal from protein	10
% kcal from carbohydrate	62
% kcal from fat	28
% kcal from saturated fat	5
Fiber (g)	23

Italicized values are less than the recommended amounts for women 31–50[15]	Micronutrient	Content	Unit
	Vitamin A (total retinol activity equivalents)	193	mcg
	Vitamin D	2.4	mcg
	Vitamin E (total alpha-tocopherol equivalents)	23	mg
	Vitamin K	86	mcg
	Vitamin C	84	mg
	Thiamin	2.1	mg
	Riboflavin	1.9	mg
	Niacin (equivalents)	35	mg
	Vitamin B6	2.7	mg
	Folate (equivalents)	1391	mcg
	Vitamin B12	2.0	mcg
	Calcium	643	mg
	Phosphorus	777	mg
	Magnesium	257	mg
	Iron	20	mg
	Zinc	12	mg
	Sodium	2952	mg
	Potassium	2732	mg
	Supplements needed to ensure adequacy relative to recommendations for woman aged 30–55 years: a multi-nutrient supplement may be necessary to ensure adequate intakes in this diet.		

Comment on vegan diet incorporating low nutrient processed foods: This diet is deficient in a greater number of micronutrients than other vegan diets, and has extremely low levels of some micronutrients. Therefore, a patient following this type of eating plan should be cautioned on the risk of multiple micronutrient deficiencies and recommended to either reduce the amount of processed food of low nutritional quality or take a daily multivitamin supplement.

Because vegan diets do not include more than small amounts of processed and refined foods of low nutritional quality, they are typically higher in fiber and lower in energy density than regular diets, and general guidelines on what types of food to consume or not consume are also useful as practical implementation tools. Table 7.2 shows typical food categories and recommended usage from a popular whole food vegan manual.[16]

EPIDEMIOLOGY OF VEGAN DIET ADHERENCE AND HEALTH: BODY MASS INDEX, CHRONIC DISEASES, AND NUTRIENT SUFFICIENCY

Compared to the dietary patterns of omnivores, those of self-reported vegans are fundamentally different: their nutrition profile is lower in energy density, saturated fat, cholesterol, and protein, and higher in unrefined carbohydrates, dietary fiber,

TABLE 7.2
General Recommendations for Plant-Based Eating
Foods to Include

Whole Plant Foods
Include unlimited amounts
of a variety of these foods
on a daily basis

Whole grains: rolled and Irish oats, brown rice, wild rice, quinoa, barley, teff, millet, wheat or spelt berries, buckwheat groats, and amaranth

Legumes (dried or canned with minimal salt): lentils, black beans, navy beans, black-eyed peas, chickpeas, kidney beans, soybeans, tempeh, green beans, peas, mung beans, fava beans, lima beans, adzuki beans, homemade veggie burgers, and more

Greens (fresh or frozen): kale, collards, spinach, chard, bok choy, lettuce, arugula, beet greens, dandelion greens, purslane, parsley, cilantro, and sprouts

Roots: potatoes, onions, sweet potatoes, leeks, carrots, daikon, burdock, radishes, turnips, beets, parsnips, garlic, and ginger

Other vegetables: summer and winter squash, celery, cabbage, Brussel sprouts, mushrooms, corn, asparagus, scallions, peppers, and tomatoes

Fruit (fresh or frozen): apples, pears, peaches, nectarines, apricots, cherries, kiwi, grapes, plums, bananas, papaya, pineapple, mango, berries, and melon

Lightly Processed
Okay to include, but use
less frequently

Plant milks (unsweetened): oat milk, almond milk, hazelnut milk, soymilk, and rice milk

Whole grain: pasta, crackers, and unsweetened breakfast cereals

Whole grain flour: whole wheat, spelt, oat, buckwheat, or gluten-free mixes, or legume flours like chickpea, fava bean

Store bought (read labels and try to minimize the added salt, sugar, and oil): tomato sauces, hummus, salsa, guacamole, and other dressings

Tofu

Richer Whole Plant Foods
Use as condiments or
ingredients only and, for
most, not necessarily
every day, because of the
high-fat content

Avocado: straight avocado and guacamole

Nuts, seeds, and spreads/butters: peanuts, almonds, cashews, pine nuts, Brazil nuts, pecans, walnuts, macadamia nuts, flaxseed, chia seed, sesame seeds/tahini, and sunflower seeds

Coconut: fresh coconut flesh, canned coconut milk, and coconut cream

Use in Cooking
These additions make food
flavorful but still healthy

Fresh and dried: herbs; fresh and powdered spices; vinegar; limited amounts of salt and sweeteners such as rice syrup, maple syrup, honey, or dates; limited amounts of miso, tamari/soy sauce, and vegetable bouillon

Treats for Special
Occasions
Remember that "special
occasions" happen
infrequently

Dessert: recipes made with lots of nuts, coconut, or added sweeteners

Drinking: plant milk by the glass—save the plant milk for use on cereal or in baking; if you are thirsty, just drink water

Source: Modified from Karlsen MC. A Plant-Based Life: Your Complete Guide to Great Food, Radiant Health, Boundless Energy, and a Better Body: AMACOM; 2016. With permission of the American Management Association.

beta-carotene, folic acid, magnesium, and vitamins C, E, and K.[11,12] Epidemiological studies report that, compared to the general population, individuals who routinely eat a vegan diet have a lower body mass index (BMI), consistent with patterns in regular consumers of lower density foods with more dietary fiber.[17] For example, in a study of Seventh-Day Adventists,[18] mean BMI was 23.6 kg/m^2, reflecting typical values for other vegan groups. Several studies also indicate that, compared to other population groups, vegans have lower cardiometabolic risk factors including blood pressure and total and low-density lipoprotein cholesterol, as well as lower rates of type 2 diabetes.[11,18,19] These benefits, however, presumably depend on the type of vegan diet that is consumed.

Additionally, vegans have statistically lower overall rates of cancers and heart disease compared with individuals consuming other dietary patterns.[20,21] Statistical power for specific kinds of cancer is lower in such studies, but vegan eating patterns are associated with significantly reduced prostate cancer (65% of individuals consuming other diets[22]) and non-significant trends for reduced breast and colorectal cancers.[23,24] While these studies are associational, and therefore cause and effect cannot be delineated, based on the intervention studies described below it is likely that the effects are due to the composition of vegan food patterns. Consistent with a broadly beneficial effect of eating patterns chosen by self-described vegans, there is a trend toward reduced all-cause mortality in vegans compared with individuals self-selecting other dietary patterns.[25]

Other benefits of vegan diets have been proposed, but the data are inconclusive at present. For example, the proposed effects on rheumatoid arthritis have not been verified in a systematic review of the literature.[26] In addition, one study suggested the potential for vegan diets to improve depression, anxiety, and work productivity,[27] but these data have not yet been replicated.

The likely beneficial effects of vegan dietary patterns on risk of cardiometabolic diseases and cancers are counterbalanced by the potential of such diets to be deficient in several important micronutrients. These risks should be considered in the context that the typical diets of omnivores can also be nutritionally inadequate if healthful eating guidelines are not followed. Nevertheless, for people who follow vegan diets, it is relatively easy to consume inadequate amounts of calcium, iron, zinc, vitamin D, and particularly vitamin B12, with one study[28] reporting that half of its vegan participants were deficient in this micronutrient. As noted by the menu examples provided, the nutritional risks of a vegan diet vary based on the specific type of eating pattern followed,[11,12,28–31] and whole food based vegan eating plans appear to be the most resilient with regard to avoiding low micronutrient levels. However, all vegan diets lack the essential omega-3 fatty acids DHA and EPA, which are primarily provided by seafood. Although DHA and EPA, which are likely important for promoting cardiovascular health[13] and slowing age-related cognitive decline,[32] can theoretically be synthesized from alpha linoleic acid (ALA), this conversion is thought to be inefficient.[13,33] This implies that regular and generous portions of ALA-rich foods, such as flaxseed and walnuts,[13,33] are important in a healthy vegan eating plan. Even so there is insufficient evidence to conclude whether higher blood levels of DHA and EPA would confer greater cardiovascular protection is already conferred by the consumption of a vegan diet typically low in these essential fatty acids.

INTERVENTION STUDIES WITH VEGAN DIETS

Intervention studies have been conducted to test a variety of potential health benefits related to vegan eating patterns. Most studies evaluating the effects on weight have reported significant weight loss relative to omnivorous diets, with the net benefit of the vegan diets in the range of 3%–4%.[3,4] Such weight loss positively impacts cardiometabolic risk factors, and a review of published studies showed that vegan diets including nuts and soy have the greatest effects on cardiometabolic risk.[34] The use of vegan diets for glycemic control in people with diabetes is more controversial, perhaps due to the high carbohydrate content of these diets. A meta-analysis of multiple diet types concluded that low-carbohydrate diets may be most beneficial for diabetes management and that more evidence is needed to determine if vegan diets should be recommended.[35]

Other intervention studies have addressed the risk factors associated with vegan eating patterns. Because of a generally low intake of calcium, vegans are at risk for bone loss and tend to have lower bone mineral density.[36] However, in intervention studies, there is a trend toward reduced rather than increased bone loss over time in vegans compared to omnivores,[31] which is consistent with the suggestion that there are protective effects of plant-based eating on bone due to the lack of endogenous acid-producing animal proteins.[37]

VULNERABLE POPULATIONS

All diets have the potential to be nutritionally suboptimal depending on the foods that are chosen, and vegan diets are no exception. Individuals who follow a vegan diet are at increased risk for deficiencies in vitamin B12, vitamin D, calcium, iron, zinc, and essential fatty acids; nutrients particularly important in vulnerable populations. Therefore, health care providers should exercise caution when recommending vegan dietary patterns for pregnant women, infants, and children, all of whom experience critical periods of development that are particularly susceptible to nutritional deficiencies. Likewise, practitioners of vegan diets should exercise caution, ensuring that they seek professional advice to make nutritionally adequate and healthy food choices and are monitored for nutritional deficiencies.

Some research[38] indicates that pregnant vegan women may be at risk of having lower birthweight infants, and the known risks of vitamin B12 and iron deficiencies[39] have the potential to cause cognitive damage in the fetus.[40] The use of supplements to prevent deficiencies is therefore particularly important for vegan women before conception and throughout pregnancy.

It also has been recognized for many years that vegan eating patterns pose special challenges for infants and children.[41] In particular, vitamin deficiencies during sensitive windows of development may have long-term effects on cognition.[42] On average, children adhering to a vegan diet are known to weigh less than the median values in growth standards[43] and have an increased risk of rickets and anemia due to nutrient shortfalls[44] and the poor absorption of calcium and iron in diets with high phytic acid content.[45] A pooled analysis of 48 studies reported that a high proportion of infants who were fed a vegan diet experienced vitamin B12 deficiency, resulting in abnormal clinical and radiological signs, including hypotonic muscles, involuntary muscle movements, apathy, cerebral atrophy, and demyelination of nerve cells, with effects that persisted at measurements made at six years of age.[46] These results indicate infants consuming vegan diets should do so under medical supervision.[47] Supervision can include emphasizing the importance of breast feeding to at least six months, minimizing micronutrient deficiencies with the use of fortified cereals, and optimizing absorption of vitamins with cooking practices, such as the use of leavened bread, fermented foods, and sprouted legumes.[48]

At the other end of the nutrition spectrum, vegan diets may have a valuable role in reducing obesity in older children. One study demonstrated that older children following a vegan diet experienced equally successful weight control compared to those following menu plans adhering to recommendations of the American Heart Association.[49] Recommendations additionally can be made for ad libitum portions for many foods included in a vegan diet, while those of traditional weight loss plans cannot.

PROS AND CONS OF VEGAN DIETS

A vegan diet is a personal decision that may be precipitated by motivating factors such as cardiovascular health, religion, or concern for animal welfare and the environment. Vegan dietary patterns can be healthy if followed very carefully with regard for potential nutritional deficiencies. Vegans who avoid refined and processed foods with low nutritional quality are also likely to lose weight without the need to log food. These advantages are offset by the real risk of nutritional deficiencies, especially for individuals who frequently eat away from home, consuming commercial foods and refined oils and sugars as part of their vegan regimen. Furthermore, some people attempting to eat as vegans may find it difficult to give up the many "typical" foods of the Western diet that have no place in a healthy vegan eating plan.

The Pros: a vegan diet is likely to cause improvements in cardiometabolic risk factors and weight if followed carefully.

Most intervention studies indicate that adherence to a general vegan, whole food vegan or raw food vegan eating plan will cause some weight loss and improvements in cardiometabolic risk factors without the need for portion control and food logging inherent in most behavioral programs for health and weight management. The high fiber content of vegan regimens that do not include significant amounts of refined or processed foods is also likely to reduce hunger and increase satiety, which is a benefit that may contribute to adherence. The move toward plant-based foods is also likely to have widespread benefits for the environment and the planet.

The Cons: a vegan diet can have a substantial risk of nutritional deficiencies and requirement for substantial changes to eating habits.

Most vegan eating plans exclude many foods that many Americans eat routinely, which means that they may be hard to sustain. Vegan diets that contain processed foods, refined oils, and sugars are likely easier to sustain than whole food or raw food vegan diets, but have substantially increased risk of nutrient deficiencies, and are therefore not recommended for sustainable health. There are major risks of vitamin B12, vitamin D, zinc, calcium, iron, and essential fatty acid deficiencies, making vegan diets healthy only if care is taken to minimize the consumption of refined and processed foods, and if supplements are consumed concurrently. The risks of permanent effects of nutrient deficiencies is considerable for pregnant mothers, infants, and young children. Elderly individuals are also at risk as they are unable to consume foods that are complex in structure and have lower rates of absorption. These subpopulations should consume vegan diets only under medical supervision and with a clear plan for micronutrient fortification.

IS A VEGAN DIET RIGHT FOR YOUR PATIENT?

Patients for whom a vegan diet is most suitable are adults who are obese or have cardiometabolic risk factors, and are willing to substantially change what they eat. These changes include giving up most or all refined and processed foods, being willing to take vitamin and mineral supplements on a regular basis, and eating a diet rich in ALA (found in flaxseed, walnuts, canola oil, and soy products) to prevent nutritional deficiencies. In return for adhering to these major dietary changes, the individual or patient is likely to lose weight and reduce their cardiometabolic risk profile. The risk of micronutrient deficiencies that have long-term negative consequences are greatest for pregnant mothers, infants, and young children, making changing to a vegan eating plan undesirable for these groups in the absence of medical supervision and motivating factors other than health.

REFERENCES

1. Le LT, Sabaté J. Beyond meatless, the health effects of vegan diets: Findings from the Adventist cohorts. *Nutrients* 2014;6(6):2131–47.
2. Euromonitor Research [Internet] 2011. [cited 2016]. Available from: http://blog.euromonitor.com/2011/08/the-war-on-meat-how-low-meat-and-no-meat-diets-are-impacting-consumer-markets.html.
3. Turner-McGrievy GM, Davidson CR, Wingard EE, Wilcox S, Frongillo EA. Comparative effectiveness of plant-based diets for weight loss: A randomized controlled trial of five different diets. *Nutrition* 2015;31(2):350–8.
4. Turner-McGrievy GM, Barnard ND, Scialli AR. A two-year randomized weight loss trial comparing a vegan diet to a more moderate low-fat diet. *Obesity* 2007;15(9):2276–81.
5. Aleksandrowicz L, Green R, Joy EJ, Smith P, Haines A. The impacts of dietary change on greenhouse gas emissions, land use, water use, and health: A systematic review. *PloS One* 2016;11(11):e0165797.
6. Mekonnen MM, Hoekstra AY. A global assessment of the water footprint of farm animal products. *Ecosystems* 2012;15(3):401–15.
7. Springmann M, Godfray HCJ, Rayner M, Scarborough P. Analysis and valuation of the health and climate change cobenefits of dietary change. *Proc Natl Acad Sci USA* 2016;113(15):4146–51.
8. Huang R-Y, Huang C-C, Hu FB, Chavarro JE. Vegetarian diets and weight reduction: A meta-analysis of randomized controlled trials. *J Gen Intern Med* 2016;31(1):109–16.
9. Ornish D, Brown SE, Billings J, Scherwitz L, Armstrong WT, Ports TA, McLanahan SM, Kirkeeide RL, Gould K, Brand R. Can lifestyle changes reverse coronary heart disease?: The lifestyle heart trial. *The Lancet* 1990;336(8708):129–33.

10. Richter CK, Skulas-Ray AC, Champagne CM, Kris-Etherton PM. Plant protein and animal proteins: Do they differentially affect cardiovascular disease risk? *Advances in Nutrition: An International Rev J* 2015;6(6):712–28.
11. Craig WJ. Health effects of vegan diets. *Am J Clin Nutr* 2009;89(5):1627S–33S.
12. Mishra S, Barnard ND, Gonzales J, Xu J, Agarwal U, Levin S. Nutrient intake in the GEICO multicenter trial: The effects of a multicomponent worksite intervention. *Eur J Clin Nutr* 2013;67(10):1066–71.
13. Davis BC, Kris-Etherton PM. Achieving optimal essential fatty acid status in vegetarians: Current knowledge and practical implications. *Am J Clin Nutr* 2003;78(3):640S–6S.
14. Barnard ND, Gloede L, Cohen J, Jenkins DJ, Turner-McGrievy G, Green AA, Ferdowsian H. A low-fat vegan diet elicits greater macronutrient changes, but is comparable in adherence and acceptability, compared with a more conventional diabetes diet among individuals with type 2 diabetes. *J Am Diet Assoc* 2009;109(2):263–72.
15. Otten JJ, Hellwig JP, Meyers LD, editors. *Dietary Reference Intakes: The Essential Guide to Nutrient Requirements*. Washington, D.C.: The National Academies Press; 2006.
16. Karlsen MC. A Plant-Based Life: Your Complete Guide to Great Food, Radiant Health, Boundless Energy, and a Better Body: AMACOM; 2016.
17. Roberts SB, Urban LE, Das SK. Effects of dietary factors on energy regulation: Consideration of multiple-versus single-dietary-factor models. *Physiol Behav* 2014;134:15–9.
18. Tonstad S, Butler T, Yan R, Fraser GE. Type of vegetarian diet, body weight, and prevalence of type 2 diabetes. *Diabetes Care* 2009;32(5):791–6.
19. Bradbury KE, Crowe FL, Appleby PN, Schmidt JA, Travis RC, Key TJ. Serum concentrations of cholesterol, apolipoprotein AI and apolipoprotein B in a total of 1694 meat-eaters, fish-eaters, vegetarians and vegans. *Eur J Clin Nutr* 2014;68(2):178–83.
20. Tantamango-Bartley Y, Jaceldo-Siegl K, Fan J, Fraser G. Vegetarian Diets and the Incidence of Cancer in a Low-risk Population. *Cancer Epidemiol Biomark Prev* 2013;22(2):286–94.
21. Fung TT, van Dam RM, Hankinson SE, Stampfer M, Willett WC, Hu FB. Low-carbohydrate diets and all-cause and cause-specific mortality: two cohort studies. *Ann Intern Med* 2010;153(5):289–98.
22. Tantamango-Bartley Y, Knutsen SF, Knutsen R, Jacobsen BK, Fan J, Beeson WL, Sabate J, Hadley D, Jaceldo-Siegl K, Penniecook J. Are strict vegetarians protected against prostate cancer? *The American J Clinical Nutrition* 2016;103(1):153–60.
23. Orlich MJ, Singh PN, Sabaté J, Fan J, Sveen L, Bennett H, Knutsen SF, Beeson WL, Jaceldo-Siegl K, Butler TL. Vegetarian dietary patterns and the risk of colorectal cancers. *JAMA Internal Med* 2015;175(5):767–76.
24. Penniecook-Sawyers JA, Jaceldo-Siegl K, Fan J, Beeson L, Knutsen S, Herring P, Fraser GE. Vegetarian dietary patterns and the risk of breast cancer in a low-risk population. *Br J Nutr* 2016;115(10):1790–7.
25. Orlich MJ, Singh PN, Sabaté J, Jaceldo-Siegl K, Fan J, Knutsen S, Beeson WL, Fraser GE. Vegetarian dietary patterns and mortality in Adventist Health Study 2. *JAMA Internal Medicine*. 2013;173(13):1230–8.
26. Hagen KB, Byfuglien MG, Falzon L, Olsen SU, Smedslund G. Dietary interventions for rheumatoid arthritis. *Cochrane Database Syst Rev* 2009;1.
27. Agarwal U, Mishra S, Xu J, Levin S, Gonzales J, Barnard ND. A multicenter randomized controlled trial of a nutrition intervention program in a multiethnic adult population in the corporate setting reduces depression and anxiety and improves quality of life: The GEICO study. *American Journal of Health Promotion* 2015;29(4):245–54.
28. Gilsing AM, Crowe FL, Lloyd-Wright Z, Sanders TA, Appleby PN, Allen NE, Key TJ. Serum concentrations of vitamin B12 and folate in British male omnivores, vegetarians and vegans: Results from a cross-sectional analysis of the EPIC-Oxford cohort study. *Eur J Clin Nutr* 2010;64(9):933–9.

29. Herrmann W, Schorr H, Obeid R, Geisel J. Vitamin B-12 status, particularly holotrans-cobalamin II and methylmalonic acid concentrations, and hyperhomocysteinemia in vegetarians. *Am J Clin Nutr* 2003;78(1):131–6.
30. Waldmann A, Koschizke JW, Leitzmann C, Hahn A. Homocysteine and cobalamin status in German vegans. *Public Health Nutr* 2004;7(03):467–72.
31. Ho-Pham L, Vu B, Lai T, Nguyen N, Nguyen T. Vegetarianism, bone loss, fracture and vitamin D: A longitudinal study in Asian vegans and non-vegans. *Eur J Clin Nutr* 2012;66(1):75–82.
32. Masana MF, Koyanagi A, Haro JM, Tyrovolas S. n-3 Fatty acids, Mediterranean diet and cognitive function in normal aging: A systematic review. *Exp Gerontol* 2017;91:39–50.
33. Sanders TA. Plant compared with marine n-3 fatty acid effects on cardiovascular risk factors and outcomes: What is the verdict? *Am J Clin Nutr* 2014;100(Supplement 1):453S–8S.
34. Ferdowsian HR, Barnard ND. Effects of plant-based diets on plasma lipids. *Am J Cardiol* 2009;104(7):947–56.
35. Ajala O, English P, Pinkney J. Systematic review and meta-analysis of different dietary approaches to the management of type 2 diabetes. *Am J Clin Nutr* 2013;97(3):505–16.
36. Ho-Pham LT, Nguyen ND, Nguyen TV. Effect of vegetarian diets on bone mineral density: A Bayesian meta-analysis. *Am J Clin Nutr* 2009;90(4):943–50.
37. Bonjour J-P. Nutritional disturbance in acid–base balance and osteoporosis: A hypothesis that disregards the essential homeostatic role of the kidney. *Br J Nutr* 2013;110(07):1168–77.
38. Mangels AR, Messina V. Considerations in planning vegan diets: Infants. *J Am Diet Assoc* 2001;101(6):670–7.
39. Piccoli G, Clari R, Vigotti F, Leone F, Attini R, Cabiddu G, Mauro G, Castelluccia N, Colombi N, Capizzi I. Vegan–vegetarian diets in pregnancy: Danger or panacea? A systematic narrative review. *BJOG: An International J Obstetrics & Gynaecology* 2015;122(5):623–33.
40. Olsen SF, Knudsen VK. Folic acid for the prevention of neural tube defects: The Danish experience. *Food Nutr Bull* 2008;29(2_suppl1):S205–S9.
41. Jacobs C, Dwyer JT. Vegetarian children: Appropriate and inappropriate diets. *Am J Clin Nutr* 1988;48(3):811–8.
42. Benton D. Vitamins and neural and cognitive developmental outcomes in children. *Proc Nutr Soc* 2012;71(01):14–26.
43. Sanders T. Growth and development of British vegan children. *Am J Clin Nutr* 1988;48(3):822–5.
44. Black MM. Micronutrient deficiencies and cognitive functioning. *J Nutr* 2003;133(11):3927S–31S.
45. Sanders T, Reddy S. Vegetarian diets and children. *Am J Clin Nutr* 1994;59(5):1176S–81S.
46. Nyaradi A, Li J, Hickling S, Foster J, Oddy WH. The role of nutrition in children's neurocognitive development, from pregnancy through childhood. *Prenatal and Childhood Nutrition: Evaluating the Neurocognitive Connections*: Apple Academic Press; 2015;35–77.
47. Fewtrell M, Bronsky J, Campoy C, Domellöf M, Embleton N, Mis NF, Hojsak I, Hulst JM, Indrio F, Lapillonne A. Complementary Feeding: A Position Paper by the European Society for Paediatric Gastroenterology, Hepatology, and Nutrition (ESPGHAN) Committee on Nutrition. *J Pediatr Gastroenterol Nutr* 2017;64(1):119–32.
48. Gibson RS, Heath A-LM, Szymlek-Gay EA. Is iron and zinc nutrition a concern for vegetarian infants and young children in industrialized countries? *Am J Clin Nutr* 2014;100(Supplement 1):459S–68S.
49. Macknin M, Kong T, Weier A, Worley S, Tang AS, Alkhouri N, Golubic M. Plant-based, no-added-fat or American Heart Association diets: Impact on cardiovascular risk in obese children with hypercholesterolemia and their parents. *J Pediatr* 2015;166(4):953–9. e3.

8 The Weight Watchers Diet

Megan Barnett

CONTENTS

OVERVIEW

Weight Watchers is the most widely used commercial diet in the world. It currently serves more than one million members who attend more than 29,000 weekly meetings in 27 countries.[17]

Weight Watchers is a paid program which promises to allow its participants to eat any foods desired, as long as they count the "point" value of the food. "Points" are used as a method of calorie counting. All foods are assigned "points" based on their caloric content, but they may be increased in foods higher in sugar or saturated fat, and decreased in foods high in protein or fiber. This is to encourage healthy choices.

The Weight Watchers program also involves some optional but commonly used tools such as a diet plan, weekly meetings for support, and tips for exercise and mindful eating. Participants pay a monthly fee that varies based on how many of the

program's tools they wish to use. If the participant chooses to attend weekly meetings, they will meet to weigh-in, discuss their weight loss progress, and will hear
a presentation about a health or diet-related topic presented by a Weight Watchers
leader.

This chapter will review Weight Watcher's history including the progression of
how their diet has changed over the years, the current program and cost, what the
current research shows, typical results that participants experience, the pros and cons
of this program, and finally, who will benefit most from this diet.

BACKGROUND

Weight Watchers was originally started by Jean Nidetch. Nidetch was born and
raised in Brooklyn where she graduated from Girl's High School. Although she
started a business administration course at City College in New York City, she was
not able to finish the course due to her father's passing. After this, she worked at a
furniture company, and later with the Internal Revenue Service (IRS). During this
employment, she met her first husband. She became a homemaker after having her
second child. During this time, she remained active with volunteer work.[9]

Jean has said that she has struggled with her weight for most of her life. She has
admitted to struggling with compulsive eating at night and despite trying many diets,
she had been unable to lose weight and keep it off.[9,18]

In 1961, Nidetch said that she had become desperate to lose weight, so she decided
to go to New York City Department of Health's Bureau of Nutrition for help. There,
she was given a strict diet, which she later used as the diet for the original Weight
Watchers program.[9]

Nidetch was unable to follow the diet without "cheating," and felt that the staff at
the clinic did not understand why she was cheating as they had never struggled with
their weight. For this reason, she decided to share the diet with six of her friends and
to start meeting with each other weekly to share their personal struggles. With these
meetings and with the support of her friends, Nidetch was able to lose 72 pounds
within one year. She was able to maintain this weight until her death in 2015.[9,17,18]

This new method of dieting with the support of and accountability to others soon
spread and many others wanted to join. When Nidetch decided to open this support up to the public, 400 people showed up for the first meeting in her apartment.
Nidetch took these people in small groups throughout the day to make sure they all
got the support they needed.[17]

After Nidetch helped Al Lippert, a local businessman, lose weight, he convinced
her to make her program into a company. In 1963, Weight Watchers became a company. After expanding, Nidetch and Lippert decided to use participants who had met
their weight goal as meeting leaders as they felt they would be able to empathize with
the participants. The program has since been expanded through franchises around
the country as well as internationally.[9]

The original Weight Watchers diet was based on the New York City Department
of Health's Bureau of Nutrition's diet plan. Later, the point system was developed,
which has also been modified over time. In 1978, exercise and behavior modification

guidelines were also added. The weekly meetings have remained an integral and mostly unchanged part of the program.[9]

Weight Watchers International was sold to the H.J. Heinz Company in 1978. Since its acquisition by Heinz, entrees, breakfasts, snacks, and desserts have been developed to be sold in supermarkets around the country. These are manufactured by the Weight Watchers Gourmet Food Company, also an affiliate of H.J. Heinz, and by licensees. These items are designed to fit into the Weight Watchers food plan and can be used by members and non-members. A number of other products and services are also offered under the Weight Watchers trademark, such as cookbooks, appointment calendars, exercise tapes, and a national magazine.[9,17]

Despite the company being sold, Nidetch remained the spokesperson for the company until 1984, when she retired. Nidetch passed away April 29, 2015, at the age of 91.[9,18]

DIET PROGRESSION

The Weight Watchers program has changed and updated their diet plans frequently since becoming a company. Overall, the plans have become more liberal over time allowing for more choices, but have maintained a moderate Caloric restriction as a goal. This section will review how the diet has changed over time.

ORIGINAL WEIGHT WATCHERS DIET PLAN

In the 1960s, the Weight Watchers diet plan was originally much more structured than today's points system. Basic rules were provided (as listed below) in addition to specific meal plans for participants to follow. Lists of "allowed" and "not allowed" foods were given for each food group to allow for some substitutions. This plan was based on the New York City Department of Health Bureau of Nutrition's diet plan as previously mentioned.

A greater appreciation of the Weight Watchers' message to participants during this era is reflected in their "10 Helpful Hints while Dieting" educational handout as listed below:[10]

1. Do not count calories. 200 calories of cake is never a substitute for a 200-calorie lunch. You can't bargain with the diet.
2. Weigh your food carefully. You'll be amazed at how much more will be on your plate when you weigh food rather than guess at its weight.
3. Carry your "before" picture and a mental image of your ideal figure with you at all times.
4. Weigh yourself once a week only. Weight can fluctuate daily for various reasons. It is the weekly average weight loss that is important. Be sure to weigh yourself at the same time each week, on the same scale, under the same conditions.
5. Take advantage of the "free" foods allowed in this diet. Never allow yourself to be hungry.

6. Be aware that you are learning new eating habits even away from home. It is possible to follow this diet plan in any restaurant anywhere in the world if you really want to.
7. Do not allow sympathetic thin friends or envious fat ones to give you "permission to deviate from your diet plan."
8. Follow the diet honestly. The key to successful weight loss and its maintenance is learning discipline and control.
9. Think before you eat. When tempted to gobble, just stop and count to ten and look at your "before" picture, remember your reasons for wanting to reduce.
10. Be patient!

1970s

In the 1970s, Weight Watchers began to expand their diet to allow for some choices. Rather than having one meal plan for everyone, three levels of diet plans were chosen from based on the participant's preference for having more or fewer choices. Lists of "legal" and "illegal" foods were provided for each food group again to allow for some substitutions, depending on which diet plan was chosen.

Participants could choose from the following plans:[11]

Full Choice Plan. This was the most liberal of the plans in that it allowed for more choices. With this plan, a sample meal plan was provided with the option to use the "legal" and "illegal" food lists to make some substitutions.

In addition to the meal plan, a number of additional servings of "bonus" and "occasional" substitutes could be added weekly.

Limited Choice Plan. This plan was not as liberal as the "full choice plan," but not as strict as the "no choice plan." This option was for participants who preferred to have more structured eating plans. This option continued to allow some substitutions from the meal plan using the "legal" and "illegal" food lists, but it provided fewer alternative choices and fewer extra options.

For this reason, this option also tended to provide fewer calories.

No Choice Plan. This plan was the most structured plan, and was intended to be used temporarily (from two days up to two weeks) to help participants to see more weight loss results more quickly, or to be used to get through weight loss plateaus. Nidetch also recommended this plan for those starting out who have more of an "urge to eat indiscriminately."

This plan offered a specific meal plan without substitutions and was the most calorie-restricted (about 1200 calories or less).[11]

1980s

During the 1980s, what were called the "Quick Start Programs" were developed. These programs introduced the use of diet exchanges to provide even more choices for participants within their meal plans. Participants would initially receive a more structured plan which offered fewer choices and calories, but the option of "exchanging" foods using lists of foods that could be exchanged for each other would be added weekly. This supported greater weight loss at the beginning followed by a maintenance-style diet plan.[12]

This plan was soon updated to what was called the "Quick Start Plus" program. This program continued with the same meal plan with the option of "exchanges," but also added the option of eating some higher fat foods, such as peanut butter, and some higher fat meats.

The rules provided for the Quick Start Programs were as follows:[12]

The Food Plan:

1. Three meals per day should be eaten. Snacks should be planned.
2. Breakfast is required with at least 1 Protein Exchange or bread with milk.
3. No more than 3 eggs per week, 4 oz of hard or semi-soft cheese, 9–12 oz fish or shellfish, and no more than 12 oz of limited (higher fat) meats should be eaten per week.

Foods that could be exchanged were provided in a list for the following groups: fruit, vegetables, fat, protein, bread, milk.

QUICK SUCCESS PROGRAM

In 1988, the Quick Success Program was developed. This program continued to use a provided meal plan with optional diet exchanges, but also added the options of using a Lacto-ovo-Vegetarian or reduced sodium (2,000 mg/day) menu. This allowed Weight Watchers to be used by people who may not have been able to in the past. The recommended vegetable intake was also increased from 2 to 3 minimum servings per day.[13]

1990s

In the 1990s, the Personal Choice program was developed. This program continued with the use of diet exchanges but sodium, cholesterol, and fat were limited in all plans. Three diet plan "levels" were created for this program with varying levels of calorie restriction. This first level was the most calorie-restricted, which was intended for more rapid weight loss at the beginning, followed by a moderately calorie-restricted diet, and finally a maintenance diet plan.[15]

In addition to providing meal plans and diet exchanges, optional daily and weekly added calorie options were also available to choose from a provided list.

In 1997, the 1-2-3 Success program introduced the "points" system of calorie counting, which continues to be used today. In this program, foods were assigned "points" based on the content of calories, fiber, and fat. Unlike the modern Weight Watchers program, a core diet plan was still provided to be followed, and the points were used in lieu of the previous diet exchanges to add variety.

2000s

The Points system has continued to evolve throughout the 2000s.

In 2004, the Turn Around program was developed. This program started the transition of using a daily allotment of points without the use of a set meal plan rather than using points only as exchanges. "Flex points" were also added, which included foods that could be eaten without using the normal daily points allotment. These included low calorie foods, beverages, and condiments.

Most recently, due to more recent research and recommendations about healthy eating, the points system has evolved to assign a higher point value to foods with added sugars and saturated fats and a lower value to foods with more fiber and protein.

The following are the current "4 Guiding Principles of Weight Watchers:"[16]

1. Any program developed by Weight Watchers must promote healthy weight loss. This translates into a program designed to:
   a. Produce a weight loss of up to an average of two pounds per week after the first three weeks (when losses may be greater due to water loss)
   b. Recommend food choices that not only are lower in calories, but also meet current scientific guidelines for optimum nutrition in order to help reduce risk for chronic disease
   c. Construct a fitness and exercise plan that provides full range of weight- and health-related benefits
   d. Maintain weight loss in which the program goes beyond advising members how to lose excess weight and addresses how to keep it off as well
2. In addition to being healthy, any Weight Watchers program must be realistic and practical, as well as liveable and flexible.
3. Weight Watchers believes in imparting knowledge about its program, rather than shrouding it in mystery. Weight Watchers promotes such understanding because it believes that members should learn not only what to do to lose weight but also why they are doing it. With this insight, people gain the confidence they need to make informed choices and to live by them.
4. Finally, again, every program created by Weight Watchers must be comprehensive. As mentioned, we do this by emphasizing changes in food intake, exercise habits, and other behaviors in a supportive environment."

2010s

BEYOND THE SCALE PROGRAM/SMARTPOINTS

More recently, the points program has been further evolved to encourage the intake of healthier options rather than being more focused on calories alone. This was done by changing the point value system to give foods high in saturated fat, sugar or sodium a higher points value, and foods high in fiber or protein a lower points value. Fruits (unless in liquid form) and vegetables continue to be point-free.

The new programs have also taken advantage of modern technology by allowing users to use their computers or smartphones to track their points. They can also use their phones and the internet to chat with other Weight Watchers users, to get access to recipes and tips, and to use a personal coach for an extra fee.

Physical activity guidelines are also provided for this program and are based on the recommendations of the American College of Sports Medicine and the American Heart Association.

Eight behavioral habits related to weight management have been identified by Weight Watchers for this program and new members are provided with a quiz to determine which behaviors they should work on. These habits are discussed at Weight Watchers meetings.[17]

HOW THE DIET WORKS

Weight Watchers diet programs have always been based on using a moderate calorie restriction for weight loss. Although the initial diets were more structured and strict with diet choices, with the diet evolving with new research to promote the intake of more protein and fiber and less sugar, saturated fat, and sodium, calorie restriction continues to be at the heart of all programs.

Although Weight Watchers has always suggested healthy balanced guidelines for members, the original points program was based on calories alone. At that time, one point was equivalent to about 50 calories. With the current program, the points value of foods are increased if they contain a significant amount of sugar or saturated fat, and are decreased if the food contains a significant amount of protein or fiber.

The daily points values are calculated based on the member's height, weight, activity level, gender, age, and goal weight with a minimal calorie level of about 1200 calories per day.

Recipes are available online and through books that can be purchased by members. Because this diet focuses on calories and not on avoiding or limiting specific foods, it can be tailored to fit alternative eating patterns, such as for vegetarian or vegan diets.

The weekly meetings have also remained an integral part of the Weight Watchers program, although it is now possible to be a remote member through purchase of online tools. The meetings are held weekly during which participants are weighed to track their progress. They will then discuss their successes and their struggles with diet in the past week with fellow members. The meeting leader also reviews a set topic about healthy lifestyles. Members have also cited meetings as a part of their success as they keep them accountable and more motivated.

Weight Watchers has recently revised their program with more of a focus on general health and body positivity, rather than on weight alone. Despite this, Weight Watchers continues to be based on calorie counting and weight loss is the ultimate goal. This program is called "Beyond the Scale."

The current Weight Watchers weight loss plan is designed for a rate of weight loss of up to two pounds per week, except for within the first three weeks at which time they may lose more than two pounds per week. Participants who are not weighed weekly at meetings are required to enter their own weights online weekly. If a participant loses weight at a greater rate, they are encouraged to review the plan guidelines and adapt them, if necessary, to avoid rapid weight loss.[17]

CURRENT WEIGHT WATCHERS PARTICIPATION RULES

Weight Watchers now requires written medical permission from a medical professional to join their meetings for children under 17 years of age. In addition, teens and
nursing women who want to attend meetings must follow a special meal plan and
policies to meet their specific requirements.[17]

Weight Watchers prohibits participation in its weight loss plan for children under
the age of 10, those individuals with an active medical diagnosis of bulimia ner-
vosa, and during pregnancy. Weight Watchers also prohibits participation from those
whose weight is less than five pounds above the minimum weight of the Weight
Watchers Weight Ranges. This range uses body mass index (BMI), with a BMI of
20 being the minimum allowed weight. Participants must provide their weight and
height before signing up, and are not allowed to continue if their BMI is 20 or lower.
Weight Watchers also prohibits subscription to their online weight loss products and
program by individuals age 18 years and younger.[17]

Participants who have medical conditions or who take medications are allowed
to use Weight Watchers, but are encouraged to share their participation with their
primary care providers.[17]

PHYSICAL ACTIVITY GUIDELINES

Participants are encouraged to exercise as a part of this program. There are no specific exercise recommendations, but participants can track their exercise to earn what
is called "FitPoints™." The Weight Watchers app has the option of syncing with
other fitness devices and apps. Weight Watchers website also offers online fitness
classes for members to use. There is also a social aspect in which participants can
participate in physical activity challenges with each other.[17]

CURRENT RESEARCH

Research has shown that the Weight Watchers' diet is equally as effective as any
calorie-restricted diet plan. Participants who are compliant with the diet have been
able to lose about 5%–10% of their weight within 12 months.[1,3,5,7,8,14] This weight
loss has been shown to be similar to other commercial programs, including Atkins,
Ornish, Slim Fast, Rosemary Conley's eat yourself slim, and Zone Diets.[2,3,5,14]

Weight Watchers has been studied for its effectiveness in weight loss as compared to self-help or regular primary care visits.[4,7,8] In the study from Jebb et al.,
standard care was defined as participants receiving weight loss advice from their
primary care practitioner.[8] The practitioners were made aware of and encouraged
to use national guidelines for healthy eating and weight loss. In the study from
Fuller et al., standard care was the same, but their practitioners were all nurses,
and there was no mention of the nurses being made aware of national weight loss
advice. The frequency of visits was up to the participant and practitioners.[4] In the
study by Heshka et al., participants were randomized to either Weight Watchers
or a self-help program. Participants in the self-help group received 20 minute con-
sultations with a dietitian at baseline and week 12. They were also given publicly

available printed materials about weight loss. Other resources such as websites, telephone numbers, and library books about weight management were also brought to their attention.[7] In these studies, participants in the Weight Watchers program did lose more weight and were able to keep weight off for a longer period of time compared to self-help or primary care visits only. In the study, participants lost twice as much weight as with standard care. Participants in standard care received weight loss advice from their primary care provider only. They were able to keep some weight off within at least two years.

In a review,[5] commercial weight loss programs with control care (no intervention, printed materials only, health educational curriculum, or <3 sessions with a provider) were compared.[5] This review found that all commercial programs showed greater weight loss after 12 months than control. Weight Watchers showed an average of 2.6% greater weight loss after 12 months than participants with control care. Attrition was reported to be variable in these trials and adherence was variable, which was similar to other commercial diets. In this review, Weight Watchers was found to have consistently greater weight loss compared to controls and participants were able to sustain beyond 12 months, but whether it is superior to behavioral counseling was unclear. Weight Watchers was also found to be one of the most cost-effective programs. This review recommended that providers only refer to Weight Watchers or Jenny Craig if referring patients to a commercial program for weight management based on their more consistent results.

Another study, performed in the United Kingdom (UK), analyzed participants' experiences and expectations of commercial weight loss programs, including Weight Watchers.[6] This study was completed with the Weight Watchers Pure Point System. Weight Watchers participants expressed enjoyment in learning nutrition related physiology and nutritional content of foods from reading food labels. They also liked being able to eat the same foods as family members and that no foods were "banned." Some participants felt that the support of the meetings was beneficial, while others did not. Participants expressed dislike in quality variability of meetings, expense of fresh produce, and time requirements for meal preparation.

Cost effectiveness of Weight Watchers versus standard care (primary care visits) was assessed in one study,[4,14] although this study was completed in Australia, UK, and Germany only and was funded by Weight Watchers corporation. This study found that Weight Watchers Diet could be cost-effective compared to seeing a primary care provider. This study also found that quality of life scores were increased for Weight Watchers participants, although this could be related to weight loss itself.

In comparison of Weight Watchers to other commercial diets, one study found that participants who were able to complete any program were able to lose the same amount of weight (about 5% body weight). They did find that compared to more restrictive diets (Atkin's, Slim Fast), more participants were able to continue with and preferred to use Weight Watchers for weight loss due to its more moderate inclusive diet plan. Participants in this study that were able to continue with any diet for 12 months were able to lose 10% of their weight.

In a study about diet quality,[19] Weight Watcher's higher carbohydrate plan (versus their higher protein plan) was found to more closely match guidelines for healthy eating.

Overall, research has shown that Weight Watchers can be an effective weight loss tool for some people to achieve a modest weight loss. When participants are able to continue with Weight Watchers for 6–12 months, they are able to achieve up to 5%–10% body weight loss. Participants who attend more weekly meetings tend to have more weight loss success.

Weight Watcher's diet plan has not been found to be any more effective than any other structured commercial diet plan, but compared to more restrictive diet plans, participants tend to be able to continue with this plan for a longer period of time.

Weight Watchers also tends to be a reasonably balanced plan compared to healthy eating guidelines, especially its higher carbohydrate plan as it allows for more fiber intake.

More research is needed for longer-term results past 12–24 months to determine how participants are able to maintain weight loss over a longer period of time. More research is also needed to assess the effectiveness of Weight Watchers for people with BMI >42.

TYPICAL RESULTS

Weight Watcher's results are comparable to most calorie-restricted diets. It does not cause as rapid a weight loss as more severely calorie-restricted diets (800–1000 calories per day), or very low carbohydrate diets, but the weight lost with the Weight Watchers seems to be more sustainable. Many participants have been able to maintain some weight loss for at least 12 months. Participants who are adherent to the diet and attending the weekly meetings have been able to maintain significant weight loss for a long period of time.

Weight Watchers seems to have greater adherence than other more restrictive diets since it allows greater flexibility in food choices and participants are able to buy traditional grocery foods. Recently, Weight Watchers has offered their own brand packaged food items that participants can consider as part of their diet.

Many also seem to value the weekly meetings, and participants who attend more meetings tend to lose more weight.

PROS AND CONS

Pros

1. The weekly meetings have been the most important and most defining part of their program. This has helped many people maintain motivation for a longer period of time, which is a common reason for weight regain.
2. Moderate Calorie Restriction. Because the Weight Watchers program offers a moderately restricted calorie diet, the diet has been more sustainable for many.
3. Weight Watchers focuses on traditional grocery store foods which allows participants to learn how to eat and choose healthy foods on their own.
4. Lifetime Membership. The Lifetime Membership is another great tool that can help participants to maintain motivation and weight loss long term.

Additionally, this stresses an important point that obesity and overweight is a chronic, relapsing disease that requires life-long management. When participants are able to reach their goal weight (by Weight Watcher's standards), then they can become Lifetime Members. These members no longer have to pay for membership as long as they maintain their weight, and they can continue to come to weekly meetings.

5. Cost Effective. Compared to other commercial programs, Weight Watchers is more cost effective than many.

CONS

1. Weight Watchers leaders are not medically trained experts in weight loss or nutrition but are Weight Watchers "graduates," which can lead to variability in the type of and quality of education provided to participants.
2. Weight Watchers does not provide one-on-one visits with registered dietitians or medical weight management providers. Without personalized counseling by an expert, some participants may not successfully lose weight because adjunct therapy such as weight loss medications, minimally invasive procedures, and/or bariatric surgery may be indicated.
3. Weight Watchers focuses on a point system and less on general appreciation of which foods are healthier options than others. This can result in frequent consumption of "low point" foods, such as highly processed, less healthy foods items like "100 caloric cookie" packages rather than fresh fruit, which may be designated as having comparable points.
4. Although Weight Watchers is a lower cost commercial diet program compared to many, it still costs a significant amount of money out-of-pocket. This can limit its availability to lower income populations. Many internet-based programs are now lower cost, although most of them do not offer weekly support and low socioeconomic status individuals may not have access to internet.
5. Although Weight Watchers does set different calorie/points goals for each person based on each person's individual calculations, the diet is not personalized based on the participant's food preferences. This would also be improved by having these participants meet with a nutrition professional.

IS THIS DIET RIGHT FOR YOUR PATIENTS?

Weight Watchers may be the diet for your patients if they have the following qualities:

1. *Value a support system.* Weight Watchers weekly meetings can be extremely helpful to those who find consistent encouragement and group support beneficial in losing or maintaining weight. The weekly meetings are Weight Watchers' foundational element of their program that has remained constant over the years.
2. *Patients who appreciate flexibility in diet options.* Weight Watchers is a moderately structured diet program in which participants are allowed to make their own diet decisions, as long as they count their daily "points."

Weight Watchers may not be the diet of choice under the following conditions:

1. *Patients who prefer a very structured eating plan.* Certain individuals prefer to have food choices made for them. If that is the case, Weight Watchers may not be the diet plan for you. Weight Watchers requires independent decision making of participants which may not be desirable to some individuals.
2. *Patients with eating disorders.* Weight Watchers has not been studied for use in those with possible eating disorders. If there is concern that an individual may have an eating disorder, any potential diet changes should be reviewed in detail with a medical professional before joining a program.
3. *Patients with complex medical histories that require a more customized diet plan.* If your patient has a medical condition requiring a special diet, such as congestive heart failure (CHF), Weight Watchers may not be a safe diet choice. Weight Watchers is based on general healthy eating principles, but does not always take into account specific medical conditions.
4. *Cost.*

REFERENCES

1. Ahern AL, Olson AD, Aston LM, Jebb SA. Weight watchers on precription: An observational study of weight change among adults referred to weight watchers by the NHS. *BMC Public Health* 2011;11:434.
2. Atallah R, Filion KB, Wakil SM, Genest J, Joseph L, Poirier P, Rinfret S, Schiffrin EL, Eisenberg MJ. Long term effects of 4 popular diets on weight loss and cardiovascular risk factors: A systematic review of randomized controlled trials. *Circ Cardiovasc Qual Outcomes* 2014;7:815–827.
3. Dansinger ML, Gleason JA, Griffith JL, Selker HP, Schaefer EJ. Comparison of the Atkins, Ornish, Weight Watchers, and Zone diets for weight loss and heart disease risk reduction: A randomized trial. *JAMA* 2005;293(1):43–53.
4. Fuller NR, Colagiuri S, Schofield D, Olson AD, Shretha R, Holzapfel C, Wolfenstetter SB. et al. A within-trial cost-effectiveness analysis of primary care referral to a commercial provider for weight loss treatment, relative to standard care-an international randomized controlled trial. *Int J Obes* 2013;37:828–834.
5. Gudzune KA, Doshi RS, Mehta AK, Chaudhry ZW, Jacobs DK, Vakil RM, Lee CJ, Bleich SN, Clark JM. Efficacy of commercial weight loss programs: An updated systemic review. *Annals of Internal Medicine* 2015;162:501–512.
6. Herriot AM, Thomas DE, Hart KH, Warren J, Truby H. A qualitative investigation of individuals' experiences and expectations before and after completing a trial of commercial weight loss programmes. *Journal of Human Nutrition and Dietetics* 2008;21:72–80.
7. Heshka S, Anderson JW, Atkinson RL, Greenway FL, Hill JO, Phinney SD, Kolotkin RL, Miller-Kovach K, Pi-Sunyer FN. Weight loss with self-help compared with a structured commercial program: A randomized trial. *JAMA* 2003;289(14):1792–1798.
8. Jebb SA, Ahern AL, Olson AD, Aston LM, Holzapfel JS, Amman-Gassner U, Simpson AE. et al. Primary care referral to a commercial provider for weight loss treatment versus standard care: A randomized controlled trial. *The Lancet* 2011;378:1485–1492.
9. McFadden RD. Jean Nidetch, a Founder of Weight Watchers, Dies at 91. 2015. Retrieved from: http://www.nytimes.com/2015/04/30/business/jean-nidetch-dies-at-91-co-founder-of-weight-watchers-and-dynamic-speaker.html?_r=0

10. Nidetch J. *Weight Watchers Cook Book*. New York, NY: Hearthside Press; 1966.
11. Nidetch J. *Weight Watchers New Program Cookbook*. New York, NY: NAL; 1978.
12. Nidetch J. *Weight Watchers Quick Start Plus Program Cookbook*. New York, NY: New American Library; 1984, 1986.
13. Nidetch J. *Weight Watchers Quick Success Program Cookbook*. New York, NY: NAL Penguin Inc; 1988.
14. Truby H, Baic S, deLooy A, Fox KR, Livingstone MBE, Logan CM, Macdonald IA, Morgan LM, Taylor MA, Millward DJ. Randomised controlled trial of four commercial weight loss programmes in the UK: Initial findings from the BBC "diet trials." *BMJ* 2006;332:1309–1314. doi:10.1136/bmj.38833.411204.80
15. Weight Watchers International. *Weight Watchers Healthy Life-Style Cookbook*. New York, NY: The Penguin Group; 1995.
16. Weight Watchers International. *Weight Watchers New Complete Cookbook: Over 500 Recipes for the healthy cook's kitchen*. 2014; pp. 9–10.
17. Weight Watchers official website. https://www.weightwatchers.com/us/
18. Nidetch J. Who Made America. Retrieved from: http://www.pbs.org/wgbh/theymadeamerica/whomade/nidetch_hi.html
19. Ma Y, Pagoto SL, Griffith JA, Merriam PA, Ockene IS, Hafner AR, Olendzki BC. A dietary quality comparison of popular weight-loss plans. *J Am Diet Assoc* 2007;107(10):1786–1791.

9 The Zone Diet

Catherine Fanning

CONTENTS

OVERVIEW

The relative impact of macronutrient distribution on energy balance and health promotion has garnered significant attention over the last several decades. Owing to a narrowed epidemiologic focus on the rising prevalence of overweight and obesity, the Zone Diet (ZD) emerged in the mid-1990s in response to the need to address and reassess the impact of diet on excess weight gain. Until recently, literature from the American Dietetic Association and the National Institutes of Health has generally espoused low-fat, high-carbohydrate diets for weight loss. Historical macronutrient recommendations by government nutrition boards and scientific panels have advocated for the allocation of 50%–60% of daily calories as carbohydrates, 10%–20% as protein, and less than 30% as fat. This advice was largely based on the belief that the intake of fat in excess was responsible for increased energy consumption and concomitant weight gain. While several meta-analyses have postulated dietary fat intake to be directly associated with obesity,[7] there remains a dearth of substantive scientific evidence to substantiate this theory.[2,21–23,25] Indeed, much to the contrary, retrospective findings affirm an inverse relationship between the decline in population-wide fat intake and the burgeoning ubiquity of obesity.[1,2,7] Tasked with satisfying palatability requirements of low-fat products, the food industry leaned on a stop-gap solution by replacing fat content with refined sugar. Doing so produced energy densities similar to that of an item's original high-fat counterpart, but with a striking epidemiologic response. This paradox spawned a body of research that called into question the implication of carbohydrate consumption on the obesity epidemic, reengaging nutrition experts in the ever-evolving battle around energy homeostasis.

In 1995, biochemist Barry Sears introduced the first iteration of the ZD, designed to investigate the expression of inflammatory genes through the prescribed intake of an explicit macronutrient ratio, a reduction in calories, and supplementation with omega-3 (ω-3) fatty acids. Conceptualizing food as medicine, the framework of the ZD was built upon the supposition that human hormonal responses and weight gain are directly related to the nutritional composition of ingested nutrients, alleging that nutritional and hormonal states are allied in their effects on metabolism.[9,24] Sears' work highlights two of the hormonal systems heavily influenced by dietary macronutrients: the insulin/glucagon axis and eicosanoids. His research explores these systems and their mediating effects on the inflammatory processes of obesity and its associated comorbidities, with the understanding that an inappropriate balance of macronutrients, particularly high glycemic load carbohydrates, has a causal and precipitous association with the inflammation that so insidiously and silently begets obesity.[4]

The body's regulatory systems were designed to effectively prevent depletion of energy stores. Insulin and glucagon are two opposing hormones working in tandem to maintain a homeostatic fuel balance. On a molecular level, beta cell pancreatic release of insulin serves as the primary regulator of carbohydrate metabolism, activating glucose uptake in muscle and fat cells, inhibiting gluconeogenesis and glucose output by the liver, stimulating glucose storage as glycogen in liver and muscle cells, and promoting lipid aggregation and storage. Acting in opposition as a counter-regulatory hormone, the pancreatic alpha cell release of glucagon responds to low blood glucose by promoting hepatic glycogen breakdown and concomitant gluconeogenesis from amino acids, adipose tissue lipolysis, and the release of the catecholamine epinephrine.[10–14,18]

Both the quantity and quality of dietary carbohydrates, and their respective influence on post-prandial glycemia, have been central to the conversation elucidating the ideal diet for body weight regulation. Since the early 1980s, carbohydrates have been defined by their glycemic index (GI), or rate of entry of glucose into the bloodstream, as measured by glycemic potency. Research has repeatedly shown low-GI foods to be beneficial for weight control by means of several well-defined mechanisms.[8,11,14] Specifically, a low-GI diet has been speculated to promote satiety, reduce meaningful fluctuations in glycemia and insulinemia, stimulate fat oxidation at the expense of carbohydrates, and even minimize declines in metabolic rate during periods of energy restriction.[10,11,14] Research exploring the metabolic mechanisms behind these phenomena maintains that the slow rate of digestion and absorption of low-GI foods promotes a longer period of gastrointestinal nutrient receptor stimulation, resulting in protracted feedback of cholecystokinin and glucagon-like peptide to the brain's hypothalamic satiety center. Beyond providing a more stable diurnal profile, lower GI diets have been shown to reduce insulin resistance and circulating insulin levels, decreasing post-prandial rebounds in free fatty acids, inflammation, and endothelial dysfunction.[14]

Conversely, research has revealed diets rich in high-GI foods to potentiate the organization of energy partitioning in a way that is conducive to body fat gain. Sears built his diet on evidence that suggests adiposity induced by high carbohydrate intake in the form of refined sugars to be a direct consequence of the diet's relative and inherent elevated GI. The typical Western, high carbohydrate diet replete with refined grains, pastries, potatoes, and bread products is digested and absorbed rapidly into the bloodstream, causing a high glycemic load (GL) and resultant heightened demand for insulin secretion. The literature suggests that diets founded on high GL foods increase post-prandial insulin levels, favoring insulin-mediated glucose oxidation and lipid deposition via rapid activation of rate-limiting enzymes. This serves to produce elevated adipose accumulation while simultaneously suppressing lipolysis through the inhibition of fatty-acid transport into the mitochondria.[8,10,11,14] Studies have effectively shown long-term consumption of these high glycemic load carbohydrates to be detrimental to health and metabolism, with chronic levels of hyperglycemia and hyperinsulinemia eliciting hormonal and physiologic changes that favor insulin resistance, appetite stimulation, and inflammation.

Sears' work explored an important, yet poorly defined potential consequence of this diet-induced hyperinsulinemia and its effect on certain metabolic fatty-acid pathways. His research focused on polyunsaturated fatty acids (PUFAs), long known for their immunomodulating capacity, influencing several inflammatory pathways through extracellular receptor interactions and intracellular signaling mediators.[15,26] The last 50 years have brought considerable attention to the role of PUFAs as precursors to specific 20-carbon PUFAs known as eicosanoids, which act as short-lived yet highly potent lipid-derived cellular mediators of cytokine production, cell signaling, hormonal regulation, and inflammation.[15–17]

With evolving understanding around eicosanoids and their production, Sears and others discovered that dietary intake of fats, specifically the 20-carbon eicosanoid precursors arachidonic (AA) and eicosapentaenoic acid (EPA), greatly influence the direction of eicosanoid pathways. Of particular importance with regard to obesity and its inflammatory effects is AA. A 20-carbon omega-6 (ω-6) conditionally essential fatty acid central to the arachidonic acid cascade, AA controls functions involving inflammation, cell growth, and activity of the central nervous system. Chiefly derived from dietary linoleic acid (LA) found in nuts, seeds, vegetable oils, and animal fats, AA has been shown to act as the precursor to pro-inflammatory eicosanoids such as certain prostaglandins, thromboxanes, and leukotrienes. Crudely, LA undergoes a preliminary transformation into γ-linolenic acid (GLA) by delta-6 desaturase. GLA is then elongated to form DGLA (20:3), a potent anti-inflammatory eicosanoid, before being acted upon by delta-5 desaturase to form AA and, subsequently, pro-inflammatory eicosanoids. Counter to this, eicosapentaenoic acid (EPA) and docosahexaenoic acid (DHA), two long-chain ω-3 PUFAs, have emerged as anti-inflammatory nutrients, specifically in their ability to competitively inhibit the conversion of AA to pro-inflammatory eicosanoids, and instead promote the proliferation of anti-inflammatory eicosanoids and their subsequent incorporation into membrane phospholipids.[15–17]

Sears helped to pioneer research proposing that the enzymes required for the synthesis of the eicosanoid precursors (DGLA, AA, and EPA) are common to both the ω-6 and ω-3 fatty acid metabolic pathways, which suggested the potential for manipulation of their enzymatic activity through dietary means. As both DGLA and EPA are substrates for the delta-5 desaturase enzyme, Sears posited that supplementation with EPA would act as a feedback inhibition, suppressing the delta-5 desaturase pathway, thereby reducing the production of AA from DGLA.[9,16,17] Alterations in plasma AA:EPA ratio have been cited as causative of dysfunction in the metabolism of obese individuals, cautiously affirming the observation that fatty acid desaturase activity serves as a biomarker for the development of obesity and its related disorders.[16,17]

According to Sears, the final piece of the eicosanoid puzzle hinges on endogenous insulin production which, in excess, is purported to substantially increase delta-5 desaturase activity, thereby promoting AA-derived pro-inflammatory eicosanoids. He contended that an appropriate, delicate balance of daily carbohydrate, protein, and fat intake was central to the maintenance of tight control over the insulin-glucagon axis and, consequently, eicosanoid formation. Recognizing the promise of eicosanoids as potential therapeutic agents against the pathophysiology of chronic disease and obesity, Sears developed the ZD not only to promote weight loss, but also to foster greater homeostatic hormonal stability.

HOW THE DIET WORKS

The ZD is based on Sears' research efforts to create a diet he posited would encourage a metabolic state of hormonal efficiency, purporting satiety, increased energy and physical performance, heightened mental focus, and productivity. Weight loss, then, becomes a passive byproduct of successful dietary adherence instead of an intended primary outcome. Similar to other low-carbohydrate diets, the ZD relies on a 40:30:30 percentage macronutrient distribution comprised of complex carbohydrates, lean proteins, and healthy fats, respectively.[9]

The ZD was the first to establish "dietary food blocks" as a simplified dietary framework that would modulate circulating GL and, consequently, the body's inflammatory processes. According to Sears, each ZD meal consists of an appropriate balance of protein (7 grams), carbohydrate (9 grams), and fat (3 grams) blocks. Sears provides participants with a ZD "block list" for ease of meal preparation, with the goal of including equal block ratios of protein, carbohydrate, and fat at each meal and snack to meet the requisite macronutrient distribution while optimizing hormonal and enzymatic control. Sears contends that the regulation of insulinemia depends not only on the glycemic load, but also on the ratio of protein to carbohydrate at each meal.[9] As research has shown, while protein is known to induce insulin secretion, it has a much more pronounced effect on the primary counter-regulatory hormone, glucagon, important for the regulation of post-prandial substrate metabolism, the restoration of blood glucose levels, and the control over satiety. Despite carbohydrate and protein having similar energy densities, research has also alluded to protein's heightened thermogenic potential and facilitation of increased energy expenditure and, consequently, weight loss.

Unlike other diets, the ZD places emphasis on the quality rather than quantity of calories, under the guise that individual nutrients impart varying inflammatory potentials. The core tenets require the participant to maintain a consistently healthful balance of eicosanoids by ingesting specific, defined proportions of macronutrients to effect a favorable insulin/glucagon response. The ZD's first essential step is to understand and calculate an individual's unique protein prescription based on anthropometric factors (weight, body fat percentage) and level of physical activity, understanding that increased activity promotes increased protein turnover. These daily protein recommendations generally fall between 1.1–2.2 g/kg fat-free body mass, and are determined by multiplying an individual's computed body fat percentage by their activity factor, which ranges from sedentary to heavy weight training.

The macronutrient block method is used to establish the desired blocks of protein per day by dividing an individual's computed protein requirement by seven (for seven grams of protein for each block), and rounding to the nearest whole number. The diet recommends spreading this protein load throughout the day into three small zone-favorable meals and two zone-favorable snacks at regularly timed intervals, with no more than four to six hours in between each meal.[9] Subsequently, the carbohydrate dose can be derived from the desired 0.75 protein to carbohydrate ratio, supplying the body with enough carbohydrate fuel to maximize energy and meet metabolic requirements while avoiding ketosis. The carbohydrate blocks are dosed on a one-to-one basis with protein to generate the desired protein-to-carbohydrate ratio. Dietary fat, an integral part of hormone production, membrane integrity and fluidity, and energy delivery comprise the remainder of the ZD.

As a visual guide, Sears recommends the division of each plate into three equal sections, whereby one third of the plate is made up of high-quality, lean protein sources, two thirds of the plate is comprised of non-starchy vegetables and select fruits with low GIs, and healthy fats are limited to the equivalent of two tablespoons. Protein sources, designed to be the size and thickness of the palm of a hand, can be chosen from turkey, fish, egg whites, low-fat cottage cheese, lean cuts of beef, and tofu. Carbohydrates are largely limited to colorful, fiber-rich vegetables and fruits, with minimal intake of selected grains. Fats are chiefly derived from "healthier" inputs, including monounsaturated sources like olive oil, fish oils, and nuts.

The diet encourages the recognition of food as a powerful drug and, essentially, as a prescription for improved health. As color is a direct correlate to phytochemical and antioxidant potential, Zone-favorable carbohydrates are defined by their variegated contributions.[9] To mitigate feelings of hunger or deprivation, Zone meals are designed around balanced intake of high quality protein, fiber-rich complex carbohydrates, and satiating healthy fats. Dieters are encouraged to maintain no more than a four to six hour window between meals, with snacks at timely intervals after breakfast and lunch to moderate the body's natural hormonal signals.

The ZD shares many components with the Mediterranean Diet, the main difference being the reduced intake of grains and starches, a deficit offset by an increased intake of non-starchy vegetables and fruits. In this respect, the ZD can be viewed as having evolved from Mediterranean influence, though with a favorable progression toward health and metabolic harmony, whereby a global reduction in GL is coupled with a tightly regulated protein-to-carbohydrate ratio to achieve improved hormonal control. In light of the emphasis on consuming a diversity of colorful fruits and vegetables, Sears reasoned the increased dietary polyphenol contribution and its relative influence over gut biology to be one of the diet's many benefits.[9,19]

The final element of the diet rests on the intake of a specific quantity and type of fat. As consistently evidenced, dietary fat is most beneficial in the form of "noninflammatory," monounsaturated sources. Sears postulated that a 30% ratio of fats would not only allow for adequate, but not excessive, caloric intake from protein and carbohydrates, but would also confer the benefits of increased satiety from epigastric release of cholecystokinin (CCK), enhanced brain function, and improved heart health, provided the fats are sourced prudently. In the development of the ZD, Sears examined enzyme systems required for the synthesis of eicosanoid precursors common to both ω-6 and ω-3 fatty acid metabolic pathways. Evidence has shown that high levels of long-chain ω-3 fatty acids, specifically EPA, act to compete with their pro-inflammatory counterparts, improving the balance of DGLA to AA.[15–17] A resultant increase in DGLA would thereby increase production of strong anti-inflammatory eicosanoids while producing a corresponding reduction in the production of strong pro-inflammatory eicosanoids. The concomitant regulation of insulin and supplementation with EPA act in tandem to control the activity of the enzyme delta-5 desaturase, thereby causing anti-inflammatory benefits that may act against obesity and its devastating comorbidities.

CURRENT RESEARCH

As with many popular diets, analytic research on the ZD has been rather limited due to variable participant attrition, dietary non-compliance, small study sample size, and difficulties in dietary tracking. The majority of the literature to date discusses the ZD in relation to other popularized diets, with respect to weight loss, anthropometric measurements, short- and long-term efficacy, cardiovascular risk, and other metabolic biomarkers.

In a randomized-controlled trial,[22] sought to compare popular weight loss diets and their relative influence on weight loss and other associated metabolic variables. Challenging the national dietary weight loss guidelines advocating energy restriction in combination with low fat and high carbohydrate, the A to Z Weight Loss Study compared four diets, three popular and one based on national guidelines. Each diet represented a range of carbohydrate intakes: Atkins (very low carbohydrate), ZD (low carbohydrate), Ornish (very high carbohydrate), and LEARN (low in fat, high in carbohydrate, based on national guidelines).

The trial included 311 free-living overweight and obese (body mass index [BMI] between 27 and 40) premenopausal women aged 25–50 years. Participants were included if their body weight was stable for at least two months and their medications were stable for the previous three months. Participants were excluded if they were pregnant, lactating, taking a weight promoting medication, or suffered from particular medical conditions (i.e., hypertension, type 1 or 2 diabetes, heart, renal or liver disease, cancer, hyperthyroidism).

Participants were randomized into four cohorts (Atkins [$n = 77$], ZD [$n = 79$], LEARN [$n = 79$], or Ornish [$n = 76$]), and were assigned 1 of 4 corresponding diet books: *Dr. Atkins' New Diet Revolution, Enter the Zone, The LEARN Manual for Weight Management* or *Eat More, Weigh Less*. After assignment of targeted weight loss goals, each group received weekly instruction for two months led by a registered dietitian (RD), where they covered chapter and topics specific to their assigned books. Dietary composition data collected through phone-administered, three-day, unannounced, 24-hour dietary recalls were analyzed using raw unadjusted means. Outcomes were assessed at months 0, 2, 6, and 12. Weight loss at 12 months was the primary outcome, while secondary measures included BMI, fasting lipid profile (low-density lipoprotein, high-density lipoprotein, non-high-density lipoprotein cholesterol, and triglyceride levels), percentage of body fat (measured by dual-energy x-ray absorptiometry), waist-hip ratio, fasting insulin and glucose levels, and blood pressure.

Neither attrition rates nor attendance of the respectively assigned classes differed significantly among diet groups. Total energy intake did not differ among diet groups at baseline or any subsequent time point ($P > 0.40$). No significant group differences were found at baseline before randomization with regard to energy from carbohydrate, fat, or protein or in grams of saturated fat or fiber.

Results were revealing for significantly greater weight loss for women randomized to the Atkins Diet group compared with the other diet groups at 12 months, particularly when compared to the ZD ($P < 0.05$). Mean 12-month weight loss was the following for: Atkins, −4.7 kg (95% confidence interval [CI], −6.3 to −3.1 kg), ZD, −1.6 kg (95% CI, −2.8 to −0.4 kg), LEARN, −2.6 kg (−3.8 to −1.3 kg), and Ornish, −2.2 kg (−3.6 to −0.8 kg). Weight loss was not statistically different among the ZD, LEARN, and Ornish groups. Of the secondary outcomes, only body mass index was statistically lower in the Atkins group compared to the other diet groups at 12 months. Parallel changes were seen in mean blood pressure levels, with Atkins producing the largest change at all time points. There were no significant differences in insulin and glucose levels among the groups. There were significant differences across each study population in diet composition beyond carbohydrate content, with protein and fat following an inverse continuum. While the relative weight lost from baseline at 12 months was small, it was significant given that even modest weight reductions have been shown to have clinically significant effects on metabolic and cardiovascular risk factors.[20,22,25]

In 2005,[27] published a study examining adherence rates and clinical efficacy for weight loss and cardiovascular risk of four popular diets: Atkins, ZD, Weight Watchers, and Ornish. The trial included 160 free-living overweight and obese (BMI 27–42) adults aged 22–72 years with at least one of the following conditions: hypertension, dyslipidemia, or fasting hyperglycemia. Exclusion criteria included unstable chronic illness, insulin therapy, clinically significant abnormalities of liver or thyroid, weight loss medication, or pregnancy.

Participants were randomized to one of four diets: Atkins (carbohydrate restriction, $n = 40$), ZD (macronutrient balance, $n = 40$), Weight Watchers (calorie restriction, $n = 40$), or Ornish (fat restriction, $n = 40$). Over the course of two months, four one-hour long, diet-specific meetings were held by a dietitian and physician to emphasize positive reinforcement for dietary changes and to discuss barriers to adherence. Recommendations pertaining to supplement use, exercise, and external support were standardized across the four treatment groups to remove confounding variables. The primary outcomes were one year changes in baseline weight and cardiac risk, and dietary adherence.

Adherence was measured in two ways: using three-day food records at baseline, 1, 2, 6, and 12 months whereby the macronutrient intake was analyzed using a computerized diet analysis program and monthly calls where participants were asked to rate their dietary adherence level during the previous 30 days on a 10-point scale. Outcome measures were assessed as baseline, 2, 6, and 12 months.

Results found modest statistically significant weight loss at one year, with no significant differences between diet groups ($P = 0.40$). Of those that completed the trial, mean (SD) weight loss at one year was: 2.1 (4.8) kg for Atkins (21 [53%] of 40 participants completed, $P = 0.009$), 3.2 (6.0) kg for ZD (26 [65%] of 40 completed,

$P = 0.02$), 3.0 (4.9) kg for Weight Watchers (26 [65%] of 40 completed, $P = 0.001$), and 3.3 (7.3) kg for Ornish (20 [50%] of 40 completed, $P = 0.007$). The amount of weight lost was associated with self-reported dietary adherence level ($r = 0.60$; $P < 0.001$), but not with diet type ($r = 0.07$; $P = 0.40$). With regard to cardiac risk factors, every treatment group significantly reduced mean low-density lipoprotein (LDL) cholesterol levels at one year with the exception of Atkins ($P = 0.07$), with the ZD seeing a meaningful 18 mg/dL reduction. Correspondingly, each group save for Ornish, ($P = 0.60$), appreciated a significant increase in mean high-density lipoprotein (HDL) cholesterol, with the ZD seeing a 5.1 mg/dL jump. At one year, none of the diet groups affected a significant change in triglyceride levels, blood pressure or fasting glucose, though the lower carbohydrate diets (Atkins and ZD) were more likely to reduce triglycerides (−66 mg/dL), diastolic blood pressure (−5.8 mm Hg), and insulin (−6.5 μIU/mL) at the two-month mark. Attrition was most often related to the perception of difficulty regarding the assigned diet or the treatment group yielding too little weight loss. Overall, each popular diet showed a modest reduction in body weight and several cardiac risk factors at one year for those individuals able to sustain a high dietary adherence level.

In a randomized-controlled trial, McAuley et al.[28] sought to compare the high-fat Atkins Diet and high-protein ZD with the conventional high-carbohydrate, high-fiber approach diet to weight loss. The trial included 96 normoglycemic, insulin-resistant overweight women (BMI > 27) aged 30–70 years. Exclusion criteria prohibited major medical conditions, current formal weight loss programs, or a strict vegetarian diet. Participants were randomized to one of three dietary interventions: a high-carbohydrate, high-fiber (HC) diet, the high-fat (HF) Atkins Diet, or the high-protein (HP) ZD.

The first eight weeks of the study were framed as a weight loss phase, which included weekly reviews and prescribed dietary advice specific to each of the three treatment groups. Weeks 8–16 followed a similar pattern of supervision but were considered a weight-maintenance phase where dietary adherence, rather than expressly weight, was challenged. The final eight weeks required participants to follow the same dietary program without any contact with the research team. There was no energy restriction during the treatment phases, and each group was advised to participate in at least 30 minutes of activity on five days each week. The primary outcome was assessed with regard to body composition (height, weight, waist circumference) along with indicators of cardiovascular (triglycerides) and diabetes (insulin) risk.

Results indicated an appreciable decrease in body weight, waist circumference, triglycerides, and insulin levels, with significantly greater reductions in the Atkins and ZD groups than in the HC group. When compared with the HC diet, the Atkins and Zone Diets were shown to produce significantly ($P < 0.01$) greater reductions in mean weight loss (Atkins −2.8 kg, ZD −2.7 kg), waist circumference (Atkins −3.5 cm, ZD −2.7 cm), and triglycerides (Atkins −0.30 mmol/L, Zone −0.22 mmol/L). LDL cholesterol decreased in individuals on the HC and Zone Diets, with levels significantly lower in the ZD group than in the Atkins group (−0.28 mmol/L, 95% CI 0.04–0.52, $P = 0.02$). Of those on the Atkins Diet, 25% showed $a > 10\%$ increase in LDL cholesterol, whereas this occurred in only 13% of subjects on the HC diet and 3% of those on the ZD. The findings suggest that a reduced-carbohydrate, higher protein diet may be the most efficacious approach to reducing the risk for cardiac disease and type 2 diabetes.

SUMMARY OF RESULTS

Results of these studies suggest that the ZD is moderately successful at producing short-term weight loss. Research from Gardner, Dansinger, and McAuley highlight the ZD as one of many active programs capable of producing a beneficial, yet modest, effect on short-term anthropometric parameters, cardiovascular risk, and other competing metabolic variables. As with the majority of weight loss trials, studies to date are limited by high participant attrition rates, dietary non-compliance, subject homogeneity, and potential for reporting bias. The three studies produced similar results with regard to effectiveness of the ZD in producing modest, parallel reductions in weight and several cardiac risk factors at 12 months when compared with other commercial weight loss programs, but only for the minority of individuals able to sustain high dietary adherence.

With specific regard to McAuley et al.,[28] it seems likely that the larger weight reductions seen in the Atkins and ZD may have been the result of reduced energy consumption rather than the preference for alternative fuel sources from altered macronutrient composition. This depressed intake is presumably in response to diet novelty, enhanced satiety from fat or protein sources or even, perhaps, the imposed monotony from dietary restriction. The fact is, ideal ratios of dietary protein, carbohydrate, and fat for adult health and weight management remain largely unknown, but likely vary depending on genetics, race, ethnicity, patient population characteristics, environment, clinical status, and baseline nutritional biomarkers.

Success with long-term weight loss remains largely contingent upon factors beyond macronutrient composition, such as improved behavioral strategies, stronger emphasis on an increased energy expenditure, structured guidance and support, and resisting challenging societal and environmental factors impeding dietary adherence. The ZD has yet to be studied in larger populations in controlled settings or with diverse populations.

PROS AND CONS

Pros

As with any weight loss program, the ZD has its advantages and disadvantages. One of the diet's main tenets is the restriction of high-glycemic foods like refined grains and sugars, to promote a consistent and moderate release of, in lieu of spikes in, levels of glucose and insulin. Avoiding generous diet-induced fluctuations in glycemia and insulinemia has been hypothesized to produce less persistent hyperinsulinemia, a metabolic state that has been shown to contribute to the development of insulin resistance and type 2 diabetes.[1,3,5]

Similar to the Mediterranean Diet design, the ZD's use of abundant fresh fruits and vegetables provides innumerable, well-founded health benefits. The dietary fiber content of these carbohydrates has been well supported in medical literature to decrease risks for cardiovascular conditions, diabetes, obesity, and certain gastrointestinal diseases, while at the same time promoting weight loss and improved cholesterol levels, lipid profiles, and insulin sensitivity.[6,8,11,19] While the average intake of fiber in both adult and pediatric populations in the United States rests at staggeringly low levels, often less than half of the USDA recommendations (14 g per 1,000 kcal), a Zone-favorable diet naturally contributes intakes meeting or even exceeding those well-defined references.

Beyond dietary fiber, the augmentation of fruit and vegetable intake on the ZD rewards the dieter with heightened exposure to rich sources of polyphenols and antioxidants. Current literature strongly associates the contribution of polyphenols to the prevention of cardiovascular diseases, cancers, osteoporosis, diabetes, and some neurodegenerative diseases.[19] While the main dietary sources of these abundant antioxidants are fruits and plant-derived beverages, some of the mainstays of a Zone-favorable diet: vegetables, whole-grain cereals, and dry legumes, also contribute to the total dietary polyphenol intake.

The ZD's recommendation to consume ω-3 fats in lieu of saturated and trans-fats serves to moderate the consumption of plaque-building, cholesterol-containing foods. As essential fatty acids, ω-3 fats are required to be consumed through diet. They are integral to the structure and function of cell membranes, hormonal regulation, vasodilation and constriction, and inflammation. As such, these potent fatty acids have been cited as protective agents against the risk of cardiovascular disease, some cancers, and trends in obesity.[19] Contrary to the typical Western diet rich with "pro-inflammatory" ω-6 fats, like those found in vegetable oils, and saturated fats, like those in meats and dairy foods, the ZD articulates the role of anti-inflammatory ω-3 fats as a proposed means of controlling inflammation and bolstering immunity, while at the same time augmenting satiety.

Unlike many popular, commercialized diets, the ZD is painted as a relatively flexible, individually tailored approach to weight loss. While low-energy diets have been shown to affect short-term weight loss, they are often found to be unsustainable long term due to high attrition rates. Rather than a program founded in restriction, the ZD delivers satiety-producing, regularly scheduled protein and fiber-rich snacks, thereby minimizing hunger and corresponding hormonal fluctuations.

The ZD sets a healthy, realistic weight-loss goal of 1–1.5 pounds per week, falling well within the National Institutes of Health's (NIH) guidelines for safe and effective weight loss. Behavioral tools like those advocated by the ZD, including food journaling and online lifestyle video tutorials, have also proven to have a successful track record in weight loss and maintenance. Sears' ZD website provides tips and tricks for successful dietary adherence, including guided explanations for navigating nutrition labels, advice while traveling, food preparation and meal ideas, descriptions of nutrient-related terminology, and tips for introducing and maintaining moderate exercise habits.

CONS

Despite the relative promising success of lower carbohydrate diets like the ZD and the Atkins Diet, it is important to consider the possibility that the weight loss produced by these diets may be attributable to other causal factors, such as overall calorie restriction. This decreased intake may be secondary to limitation in food choices by curtailing carbohydrate consumption or to the satiating effect of providing high-protein loads. Furthermore, part of the initial weight loss may be explained by a depletion in glycogen stores from the liver and muscle, and associated reduction in glycogen-bound water lost through urine.

There has been a dearth of substantive evidence corroborating the benefits of eating a certain ratio of carbohydrate, protein, and fat expressly for weight loss. Despite claims that higher protein loads and concomitantly lower intakes of certain carbohydrate foods produce a hyper-thermogenic effect, discrepant findings persist. Additionally, while the assertion has been made and evidenced in studies that high-GI carbohydrates promote insulin release, fat storage, and the consequential propensity towards obesity, a concrete causal relationship has yet to be determined. That glycemic load is influenced by dietary factors like protein, fiber, and fat has turned the focus for the current management of overweight and obesity away from glycemic index and towards the promotion of an overall healthful balance of complex carbohydrate foods.

On the practical side, the ZD involves rigor, planning and, potentially, high food costs. Requiring daily food measuring and macronutrient counting to ensure diet loyalty, following the ZD can be relatively time consuming and tedious, necessitating the majority of meals to be prepared from scratch. Meal timing to remain in "The Zone" also proves problematic for those with busy work schedules who cannot plan to eat every couple of hours throughout the day. While the diet advocates an otherwise beneficial increase in daily vegetables, certain fruits, and whole grains, and a complementary tendency toward lean proteins and healthful fats, the cost of these foods may serve as a deterrent, especially for the low socioeconomic population where obesity often pervades.

The diet itself, while relatively uncomplicated in application, may seem intimidating or overwhelming for the average individual looking to follow an easy roadmap or meal plan for weight loss. The macronutrient meal blocks require a good deal of commitment to detail in order to guarantee the appropriate balance of nutrients at each meal, which can prove exhausting. Despite offering adequate protein, fiber, and fat as satiating elements, the ZD provides a relatively low ceiling of daily calories, which may encourage weight cycling, making it difficult to sustain long term.

Despite its inherent limitations, the ZD nevertheless presents as a viable weight loss strategy, one that removes the focus from the scale and instead places emphasis on the consumption of wholesome, balanced meals rich with vegetables, lean proteins, and healthy fats. The precise macronutrient ratio offers a concrete, albeit rigid, method of meal partitioning in an effort to foster a healthier metabolic milieu in a current food culture steeped in calorie and macronutrient imbalance.

IS THIS DIET RIGHT FOR YOUR PATIENTS?

Though not flawless, the ZD offers an individually tailored, moderately flexible approach to weight loss. For patients who have the ability to eat several small meals throughout the day, this diet is a good option. For those patients who do not enjoy calorie counting, the ZD offers a diet plan focused on moderation, specifically on macronutrient ratio rather than total daily calories. For those with inflammatory conditions, such as rheumatoid arthritis, this diet may be appealing because of its inherent focus on anti-inflammatory foods. However, it is not clear whether following this type of diet leads to a long-term positive impact on weight, lipid, and insulin markers.

Similar to many weight-loss diets, the ZD is not recommended for individuals who are pregnant or lactating as it is unlikely to meet the caloric and nutritional needs required for fetal growth and maternal health. Owing to the diet's comparatively high-protein allotment, the ZD is also not recommended for individuals with kidney disease. Evidence has shown that dietary protein intake can modulate renal function through increased glomerular pressure and hyper-filtration, amounting to a diminished glomerular filtration rate and resultant buildup of the toxic waste products creatinine and urea.[13,25] However, there are no documented reports in the literature of high-protein diets causing renal dysfunction in populations at risk for kidney disease, like those with dyslipidemia, obesity, or hypertension.

At the end of the day, dietary adherence can be influenced by a variety of inputs: socio-demographic factors (age, sex, marital status), cost, frustration in the setting of dietary restriction, limited social and emotional support, feelings of inconvenience, and difficulty observing the diet in social settings. As such, it is as important for clinicians to recognize the need for dietary weight loss programs that are easy to follow, and to understand each individual's potential barriers to adherence. As a practitioner, it is vital to assess not only an individual's clinical picture but also the many other contributing factors to the success of any weight loss program.

REFERENCES

1. Ota T. Obesity-induced inflammation and insulin resistance. *Front Endocrinol* 2014;5:204.
2. Calder P. The relationship between the fatty acid composition of immune cells and their function. *Prostaglandins Leukot Essent Fatty Acids* 2008 Sep–Nov;79(3–5):101–8.
3. Lumeng, C, Saltiel, A. Inflammatory links between obesity and metabolic disease. *J Clin Invest* 2011 Jun;121(6):2111–7.
4. Khan S. et al. Unraveling the complex relationship triad between lipids, obesity, and inflammation. *Mediators Inflamm* 2014;28;2014.
5. Ludwig, D. Physiological mechanisms relating to obesity, diabetes, and cardiovascular disease. *JAMA* 2002 May 8;287(18):2414–23.
6. Cordain L. et al. Origins and evolution of the Western diet: Health implications for the twenty-first century. *Am J Clin Nutr* 2005;81:341–54.
7. Simopoulos A. An increase in the omega-6/omega-3 fatty acid ratio increases the risk for obesity. *Nutrients* 2016 Mar;8(3):128.
8. Dumesnil, J. et al. Effect of a low-glycaemic index–low-fat–high protein diet on the atherogenic metabolic risk profile of abdominally obese men. *Br J Nutr* 2001 Nov;86(5):557–68.
9. Sears B, Stacey Bell. The zone diet: An anti-inflammatory, low glycemic-load diet. *Metab Syndr Relat Disord* 2004;2.1:24–38.
10. Markovic T, Jenkins A, Campbell L, Furler S, Kraegen E, Chisholm D. The determinants of glycemic responses to diet restriction and weight loss in obesity and NIDDM. *Diabetes Care* 1998;21:687–94.

11. Buyken, A. et al. Association between carbohydrate quality and inflammatory markers: Systematic review of observational and interventional studies. *Am J Clin Nutr* 2014;99(4):813–33.
12. Eckel R. et al. Obesity and type 2 diabetes: What can be unified and what needs to be individualized? *Diabetes Care* 2011;34:1424–30.
13. Bravata D. et al. Efficacy and safety of low-carbohydrate diets. *JAMA* April 9, 2003;289(14):1837–50.
14. Radulian, G. Metabolic effects of low glycaemic index diets. *Nutr J* 2009;8:5.
15. Lee J. Fatty acid desaturases, polyunsaturated fatty acid regulation, and biotechnological advances. *Nutrients* 2016 Jan 4;8(1):pii: E23.
16. Granstrom E. The arachidonic acid cascade. The prostaglandins, thromboxanes and leukotrienes. *Inflammation* 1984 Jun;8(Suppl):S15–25.
17. Bézard J. et al. The metabolism and availability of essential fatty acids in animal and human tissues. *Reproduction Nutrition Development, EDP Sciences* 1994;34(6):539–68.
18. Claessens, M. Glucagon and insulin responses after ingestion of different amounts of intact and hydrolysed proteins. *Br J Nutr* 2008 Jul;100(1):61–9.
19. Cheynier V. Polyphenols in foods are more complex than often thought. *Am J Clin Nutr* 2005 Jan;81(1 Suppl):223S–9S.
20. Atallah R. et al. Long-term effects of 4 popular diets on weight loss and cardiovascular risk factors. *Circ Cardiovasc Qual Outcomes* 2014;7:815–27.
21. Cheuvront SM. The zone diet phenomenon: A closer look at the science behind the claims. *J Am Coll Nutr* 2003;22(1):9–17.
22. Gardner CD et al. Comparison of the Atkins, Zone, Ornish, and LEARN diets for change in weight and related risk factors among overweight premenopausal women: The A TO Z weight loss study: A randomized trial. *JAMA* 2007;297(9):969–77.
23. Fontani G et al. Blood profiles, body fat and mood state in healthy subjects on different diets supplemented with Omega-3 polyunsaturated fatty acids. *European Journal of Clinical Investigation* 2005;35:499–507.
24. Sears B, Bell S. The zone diet: An anti-inflammatory, low glycemic-load diet. *Metabolic Syndrome and Related Disorders* 2004;2:24–38.
25. Souza R. et al. Alternatives for macronutrient intake and chronic disease: A comparison of the OmniHeart diets with popular diets and with dietary recommendations. *Am J Clin Nutr* 2008;88:1–11.
26. Luca C, Olefsky J. Inflammation and insulin resistance. *FEBS Letters* 2008;582:97–105.
27. Dansinger ML. et al. Comparison of the Atkins, Zone, Ornish, and LEARN diets for weight loss and heart disease risk reduction. *JAMA* 2005;293(1):43–53.
28. McAuley. et al. Comparison of high-fat and high-protein diets with a high-carbohydrate diet in insulin-resistant obese women. *Diabetologia.* 2005;48(5):1033.

Index